ENDORSEMENT

Food Does Make a Difference, A Beginner's Guide to Better Health
is written by Suzanne Stevens, a graduate of the Institute for
Integrative Nutrition, where they completed our cutting edge
curriculum in nutrition and health coaching taught by the world's
leading experts in health and wellness. We recommend you read this
book and be in touch with Suzanne to see how she can help you
successfully achieve your goals.
– Institute for Integrative Nutrition® (IIN)

REVIEWS

"Wonderful work and many delicious recipes for your health and well being."
— Dr. Robert O. Young, CPT, MSc. DSc, PhD, Naturopathic Practitioner, Author

"Suzanne's story is nothing short of inspiring. There is an epidemic of the so-called "Western Diseases" all around us. These diseases are incurable, debilitating, both mental and physical. Most of us reading this story are reading it because we either suffer from one of these illnesses or know someone who does. I think most of us suspect it is food related but . . . what to eat? Suzanne did more than suspect. She investigated the problem for herself and her son, and then followed through. The following through part is the hard part.

Staying with healing food is difficult to say the least. It's tirelessly swimming against the current. The media, the medical profession, your family and neighbors all tell you it doesn't matter what you eat. Buying pure ingredients is not only expensive but very hard. Learning about ingredients and finding them, shopping, cooking everything from scratch all takes time, lots of time. Start reading labels and you quickly find chicken and pork are often saturated in flavor enhancers, cream and cottage cheese have more than cream and milk, and that healthy soup has more chemicals than real flavor.

Suzanne's story is one of courage and tenacity. It inspires me to keep going and hope that I, too, can become healthy."
— Solveig Quass, Mother, Lawyer, Entrepreneur

"I can't think of a more easy and relieving way to get a better body. Thank you forever!"   —Lana Stevens, College Student

"I enjoyed following the author's progress as she researched how one's body can maintain its own health by avoiding food additives, chemicals, and some prescription medicines. In her journey to learn that *Food DOES Make a Difference*, she explains how she also learned there is often a need for emotional healing in order to improve one's physical health. The process of healing one's body is not necessarily an easy fix since it usually means we need to re-learn that our preference and love for certain foods may also be to our body's detriment."
—Edye Mitchell, Mother/Grandmother, CNS Hospice Volunteer, Retired from WIU (Western Illinois University)

AWARD

Winner of the Launch Your Dream Book Top 10 Author Contest, class of May 2018! Advanced course of the Institute for Integrative Nutrition® (IIN).

Food **Does** Make a Difference

Difference

A Beginner's Guide to Better Health

SUZANNE STEVENS

Food **Does** Make a Difference
A Beginner's Guide to Better Health

Copyright © 2018 by Suzanne Stevens

For information, contact Suzanne Stevens at www.SuzyCooking.com.

Edited by: Renee Stevens and Ashley Stevens

Cover by: Suzanne Stevens

Cover Photo from MaxPixel.net

Printed in the United States of America

ISBN: 9781729424681

DEDICATION

To all those who want to be healthy yet don't know where to begin or what to eat.

CONTENTS

ACKNOWLEDGMENTS

For my family who took this journey with me and still love me:
Robert, Andrew, Tyler, Ashley, Wesley, Lana, Jesse, and Laura.
I love you.

My husband, Robert, who encouraged me to write a book when I
never in my life considered doing so.

My mothers, father, siblings, and friends that supported me during
my transformation even though they may have thought I was
extreme.

All those people who I was led to by God that helped change my life
by what I ate and thought.

For the recipe book author's that gave me permission to use their
delicious recipes in this book.

To my awesome editors, proofreaders, reviewers and family who
helped with the flow and design of this book. Their help was
invaluable.

PREFACE

Congratulations! You have taken the first step to better health.

In my own experience transitioning to better health and as an Integrative Nutrition Health Coach, small changes propel people to make lasting changes as well as learning. I found the more I continued to learn as I was changing, the easier it was to keep on that path. When days were tough it reminded me **why** I was doing this.

I wrote this book to help you succeed in your own desires for better health. Its purpose is to give you a way that may help you attain maintainable success. So if you are tired of being sick and trying many different ways to improve your health, Or, if you need help with transitioning to health and vitality keep reading.

It **does** matter what you put into your mouth. It's time to take your health into your own hands! Be partners with your doctor.

INTRODUCTION

Change can be difficult and frightening. There are specific times in our lives when we are at a crossroad. What is the best route to take? It may be hard to know what to do, however, you have to make the decision.

One of my crossroads happened after attending lectures on different types of emergencies, the state of our nation, and how to be prepared. I planned for these and other types of emergencies, by purchasing extra food, water, personal care items, and things I use on a daily or monthly basis.

I was on prescription omeprazole at the time, and my doctor said I would be lucky if I could get a two month supply. I began to be concerned and to think about it often when I had the thought: "Do I need to be on the drug?" This thought impacted me so much it was the turning point of my transformation to a healthier life and healing my acid reflux.

HOW TO USE THIS BOOK

Section 1: Read my transformation story to help you discover that you are not alone.

Section 2: The ten steps I have found that help people change from diet to lifestyle. Take each step as quickly or as slowly as you feel ready to do so or go back to a previous step if necessary.

Section 3: Recipes to help you through transformation and to get you started.

You don't have to be perfect, you just need to get started on the right road. Keep in mind the reason you want change in your life. It will keep you focused and moving forward when you get discouraged.

Remember, it is not about what you *cannot* eat but what you *can*.

Let's get started!

Section 1

My story

MY LEARNING CURVE

It was February of 2007; our fifth child was six years old. I had a loud thought tell me that someone was missing in our family. Questioning the thought, I said to myself if it is true I would need to get pregnant soon. I was turning 40 the next month. So I decided to pray about the decision to have more kids. My answer was yes. I did not want the next child to grow up alone and so we had two. During pregnancy number six I had a bad case of acid reflux. My doctor said to take Tums and it helped. Every time stomach acid would come up, I ate them. You would have thought I was eating candy. I thought about asking my doctor about medicine for it but I never inquired about it.

My second problem was my esophagus would tighten or spasm at the chest above the sternum, closing off so much that spit wouldn't even be able to go down and it was very frightening. It happened when I ate, although it was not consistent. The only way to find relief was to throw up. This would happen at least once a month, maybe more. After giving birth to my son Jesse (number six), those health problems went away.

Six months later I was pregnant with baby number seven. As the pregnancy progressed, the acid reflux and the tightening returned (My holistic doctor told me they were actually muscle spasms). I ate the Tums when the stomach acid would come up and suffered during the esophagus tightening. Even though it was miserable, the Tums helped so I did not pursue other treatments. After the birth of my daughter Laura (number seven), both health problems did not go away.

When my baby girl was two months old, my friend Emily gave me a recommendation of a certain gastrologist. I had an endoscopy, which is a nonsurgical procedure used to examine the digestive tract using an endoscope (a flexible tube with a light and camera attached to it). The doctor was able to view pictures of my digestive tract on a monitor. He also performed an esophageal dilation or ballooned my esophagus to help with the spasms. Then he prescribed omeprazole —an acid inhibitor. I also inclined my bed. At this time the medication was prescription only. I thought nothing of it and followed his recommendation. Feeling perfectly fine, I went for a checkup a few months later, and he told me to keep taking the medicine. I had complete trust in my doctor. I asked questions; however, I nearly always followed the doctor's direction. Symptom-free and happy, I continued that way for the next two years. I was feeling good and had no reason to question. I trusted the doctor knew what was best for me. It did not occur to me that there were alternatives.

As my association with Emily increased, I got to know her health issues and struggles, including the foods she could not eat. When she ate foods that triggered her asthma, she would not be able to get out of bed and needed to use her inhaler, as well as other things that I can't recall for the next day or two. Somehow she felt the piece of cheesecake (or whatever food she had eaten) was worth the pain it caused her. I noticed how she ate and she would be excited to show me the smoothies and meals she made. It was all interesting, nonetheless, I kept eating and living each day as I did before. Why, because I felt I was healthy.

Emily would talk to me about her doctors and about what she was trying to figure out her own health. Later I was somehow prompted to make an appointment with her holistic doctor near our home. I also thought it would be good to see a natural or holistic doctor and was happy to know she had a professional medical background. I had no idea what I was going to see the doctor for. New patient visits were two months out so I thought by then, maybe I would need to see a doctor.

I was (and still am) into emergency preparedness: being ready for any type of emergency like an earthquake, power failure, or even losing a job. I purchased extra food, water, personal care items, and things I used on a daily or monthly basis. I excitedly attended lectures on different types of emergencies, on the state of our nation, and how we could be prepared for an emergency. I also taught classes to people in my community on what to store in their home for an emergency, and I organized group purchases for raw honey, water storage, wheat, and other things. It was during this time I began to consider my need to have at least a six-month supply of omeprazole. Since it was only prescription at the time my doctor said I would be lucky if I could get a two-month supply. I began to be concerned and I thought about it often when I had the thought, "Do I need to be on the drug?" Right then and there, I knew what I was going to talk to the holistic doctor about. This was a turning point in my thought process. I wrote all my questions down about myself and my children plus other things. I was ready and excited for my appointment.

Have you had a time when you had an epiphany? Something that changed your whole perspective on your life or health?

March 2011 arrived and I went to my appointment. Dr. Diane Farley-Jones was wonderful, sitting with me and answering all of my questions. I was right—she told me that I should not be on omeprazole for such a long period of time (at this point, it had been two years). She said she would help me slowly get off the medication by giving me food and supplement suggestions. When she mentioned organic produce, I felt like most people do, that organic food costs too much. She asked me to look at the prices between conventional and organic, which I did, and I noticed that organic was not that much more expensive and sometimes the same price. However, she felt that cucumbers, celery, lettuce, and apples were the most important to purchase organic. I began there and followed her suggestions with food and supplements, as I started to reduce the amount of omeprazole I was taking.

Following her advice was short-lived; I ended up not doing much at all: taking the supplements when I remembered, only shopping a little differently.

Either before or after my appointment with Dr. Farley-Jones, my friend Anne gave me a book to borrow called *Salt: Your Way to Health* by David Brownstein, M.D. He talked about why salt is the most misunderstood nutrient and how adding the right salt can help many health problems. Dr. Brownstein explained the toxicity of refined salt, the difference between unrefined and refined salt, how the right kind of salt can balance and replenish minerals, plus much more. I was encouraged by Anne since she changed the foods she ate forty years ago when discovering that refined sugar was the cause of her varicose veins. She told me this book was a good start. The book made an impact to my changing what I put into my mouth. I was astonished at what I learned and then tried for myself. I changed my salt to the brand *Real Salt* and was so amazed that the difference in the flavor of the food was sweeter and more flavorful. I was shocked about what was being given to us at the grocery store. My senses began to change.

On June 10, 2011, I had a foot operation and lots of time to read. During one of the lectures I went to previously, I was introduced to the post-apocalyptic novel *One Second After* and decided to read it. I was alarmed about what could happen during an extreme emergency. It made me think about my health again and decided that if I was truly serious, then I would follow the doctor's suggestions. I began to

take the supplements consistently and made a follow-up
appointment. It was slow going at first, although I began to read
about health and nutrition online, including learning about what
ingredients were bad for you.

It was late August 2011, we lost our home in a short sale. It was a
rough time, we had no money to rent a place to live because they
wanted a deposit, first and last month's rent. A wonderful friend took
us in so we could save money. Since she had room in her basement
we had a place to sleep. It was also close to my children's high school
so they could have some feeling of normalcy.

When life began to settle down a bit, I was eager to continue what I
was learning and did what I could. A month or so later, I had another
follow-up appointment scheduled. During this time I kept thinking a
lot about a blessing I had received from a priesthood holder in my
church (The Church of Jesus Christ of Latter-Day Saints),
encouraging me to study my church's religious document the *Word of
Wisdom* (a code of health dealing primarily with human nutrition) and
to know what was good and not good for me and to ponder the
promised blessings. One day, I was in a bulk buy shop and I saw they
had a book called *Word of Wisdom: A Modern Interpretation* by John A.
and Leah D. Widstoe, which I bought. The timing was perfect.
Another step to my learning and being directed by God for my
health.

I read every page of the *Word of Wisdom* book with earnest. The in-
depth explanations of each section of the *Word of Wisdom* were very
enlightening. I began to cook more whole foods or less pre-packaged
foods and to change the boxed cereals and snacks from regular
grocery stores to healthier options at the health food store. I would
also eat a large plateful of chicken stir-fry with a ton of vegetables
with brown rice. After an hour or two, I would begin to get really

hungry again. So I ate more. I realized later that it must have been because my body was shifting and needed the nutrition I was feeding it.

I was learning so much about things that I had never even thought about before — it was exhilarating. I was so excited about what I was learning and yet so distraught. Learning about ingredients caused me to read food labels on every item. It would make me so sick that my head and heart would hurt and caused heavy brain fog. It was so bad I even had a hard time seeing the labels I was reading. I could not believe what was in our food and why the food industry would be feeding us these things. It was at this point I realized that food does make a difference. I knew I needed to eat for strength, life, and energy, though I had no idea it could make us sick or well. Or that it really mattered what I ate. To me, it was all food.

When have you felt you were directed?

One day I was driving by Costco and I had the thought I should go in even though I was not planning on grocery shopping that day. I thought "Why not?" Since it had just opened, it was quiet as I began shopping. I passed by the book section and I met Caleb Warnock doing a book signing for his book *The Forgotten Skills of Self-Sufficiency Used by the Mormon Pioneers*. I spent time talking with him about his book and he invited me to a free class that he and Melissa Richardson (*The Bread Geek*) were teaching the following Saturday. At the class, he taught about gardening, seeds, what you can plant in the winter, and gave us a tour of his garden. Melissa taught us how to make real sourdough bread using natural yeast. I had no idea that the type of yeast could make difference in our bodies. I learned a lot of new information from Caleb's explanation on seeds and gardening which included GMO seeds, how he was trying to bring back heirloom seeds, and how he was trying to find seeds that could grow through the winter.

Caleb Warnock and Melissa Richardson were in the process of writing a recipe book *The Art of Baking with Natural Yeast*. Since it was not finished, they sold a sample version with a Danish dough whisk and a "natural yeast starter" to make my own sourdough breads (a starter contains several bacteria and yeast strains that helps the bread to rise). I purchased a few of them for family and friends I was eager to share my new knowledge with.

In November 2011 I visited my doctor again. She was pleased with my improvements. During this visit I talked to her about my son who had dryness around his nose and earlobes. She thought it might be allergies and suggested he take an electrodermal test which they had available in their office. So, I set up an appointment on December 1, 2011. I decided that the test would be good for me as well. After taking the test, it showed the types of foods he might be sensitive to, as well as checking organs and tissues for stresses. The information was interesting and the list of foods we were sensitive to was long. I decided to not eat anything on my list right then and there. In doing so, I began to feel better and my son noticed the same.

These steps really threw me into a learning spree. It also seemed that my community was in the same mode. There were many classes about health and wellness, and I went to as many as possible. I bought nearly a dozen books. Sometimes I would turn on a local radio talk station and I would have confirmation to what I was studying. One particular time was an interview with Raymond Francis, a chemist and a graduate of MIT, titled *The Cure to Obamacare* which discussed that there is only one disease (malfunctioning cells), only two causes of disease (deficiency and toxicity), and other extremely interesting information. I bought two of his books *Never*

Fear Cancer Again: How to Prevent and Reverse Cancer and *Never Be Sick Again.*

Everything I learned felt right, especially after I began to put what I learned into practice. Eating less store prepared foods, drinking raw milk, using herbs for illness, and having fewer chemicals in my home. Each class gave me a new piece of information to help me take back my health.

"Hungry for Change" is a movie from *FoodMatters.com* that also opened my eyes to what was happening in the food industry and how marketing is the drive to what is put onto our shelves. There were interviews with doctors and scientists explaining the effect chemicals and food had on our bodies and how what we ate could prove to be for our benefit or detriment. I watched other videos and read articles they had and learned more about health and wellness.

From Mike Adams, at *NaturalNews.com* I learned about our current Western food system. He has a lot of information relating to food and health which helped expand my thinking. *The pH Miracle* book taught me how our body functions best in an alkaline state, in sickness, and in health. Dr. Robert Young and his wife Shelley (authors of *The pH Miracle*) said, "Healthy bodies are not overweight or underweight. A healthy body naturally maintains its own ideal weight." I would recall that phrase during the next few years when I would gain weight after adding a new healing modality. I learned a lot from many people online and from books like *The Raw Family, The Green Smoothie Girl, Dr. Mercola, The China Study, Dr. Brownstein, FoodMatters.com, Jonathan Landsman, Western Price Foundation* and many others. Over the next few years, I watched and listened to several webinars on all kinds of subjects like thyroid health, cancer, eye health, breast cancer, oral health, and others, even if I did not have the illness they were talking about. I soon became empowered and it felt wonderful.

Are you wanting to take that step right now?

In February 2012 we were finally able to get into our own place following the short sale of our home and living in the basement of two friends' homes. I began to purge my pantry and food storage. I sold, gave away, returned boxes and cans back to a local store, even threw some food storage away. I had spent a lot of money in gathering those food items, though due to my newfound knowledge I did not want to eat that food anymore. I did the same with my medicine cabinet. I read labels and threw out everything. Then I repopulated it with more natural foods. I did not feel sad I was losing the money I had spent; I was moving forward to a healthier me.

I continued to have an awakening within me. I had regular visits with my holistic doctor and continued with her assistance to help me get off omeprazole. I appreciated her willingness to answer my questions about what I was learning, nutrition, and other ways to assist our bodies when sick. Over the next several months, eagerly learning and attending classes, I added natural remedies to improve what my family and I deserved: our health.

By April 2012 I began to eat more and more vegetarian. At one point, we only ate meat every three months. The foods we cooked, especially vegetables, were tasting so much better than before. Even some vegetables I did not like previously tasted better. I could not believe it. Was it from the elimination of refined sugars from our diet?

As I became more familiar with the produce section of the grocery store, I did notice that organic produce was not as expensive and was sometimes close to or cheaper than the price of conventional produce. I had to shop at a few different stores to get a variety of good pricing on organic produce, meats, milk, and any boxed foods I was buying. It did take more time, at first, although I became acquainted with where I needed to shop for certain items.

I began learning that if I eat well today, I would not have the common ailments related to old age. John Robbins, of the *Food Revolution Network*, is a perfect example. He is seventy years old and is very active plus he hosts retreats with his son.

What do you think about taking your health into your own hands?

On May 16, 2012, my mother was told she had lobular breast cancer. We talked and I brought her all the books I felt would help in her decision to what she to do. She decided she did not want to be sick all the time and to try healing naturally. I was now not only studying health for myself, and my son, but for my mother as well. I was seeing improvement in myself and felt she could benefit also.

Even though I was feeling better, the tightening at my chest did not go away. My mother was seeing a doctor in the same office as mine. She felt her doctor could help me. I asked my doctor about it and she consulted with my mother's doctor and found he could help me. My kind mother paid for these visits, which only took three. It turned out I had a hiatal hernia, which is when the upper stomach pushes into the diaphragm and is usually detected through x-ray - I had never had one done. At my first visit, he adjusted the stomach and sphincter (which is called an Upper Esophageal Sphincter, located at the end of the pharynx, where it protects the entrance to the esophagus) in place by pushing down fast and hard, starting at the bottom of my sternum toward my stomach. It was painful. During the next couple of weeks until my return visit, I did notice an improvement: less acid was coming into my esophagus.

During the second, visit he adjusted the stomach and sphincter the same way, which was less painful the second time, and even less painful on the third visit. During that last visit, I asked if I would be able to adjust it myself, thinking I could save my mother money. He said my stomach is where it should be so I would be pushing the sphincter back into place. Then taught me how to do it. He told me to bend my thumb and to insert the knuckle at the bottom of my sternum and push down as often as I needed to. I did that several times a day for several months. One day, I realized that I did not have to do it anymore. It was fixed.

It was during my second visit that I was exposed to the idea that emotions played a part in disease. I don't remember the precise details, yet he talked me through my emotions surrounding my parents' divorce. It was painful because I did not want them to get divorced but they did. The stress of the situation was held in my stomach, contributing to my acid reflux. He worked with me to forgive them and allow myself to be okay with it, even though I was not. Looking back, this exposure to emotional healing was good because when I was ready to dive deeper into this type of healing, I was already familiar with it.

My grandmother also dealt with acid reflux and a hiatal hernia for many years. Again, I was amazed how easily such a thing could have been healed. How would anyone ever know unless they were looking for alternatives and having people direct them to others who may be able to help? Later, I found out I had all three types of acid reflux—1. Typical acid reflux, or acid coming up the esophagus; 2. A hiatal hernia; and 3. Tightening in the esophagus which may have been caused by the acid. Since my hiatal hernia was better there was hope for healing the other two problems.

By mid-2012 I was completely off omeprazole. I may have gotten off it too fast because, after one of my visits, Dr. Farley-Jones mentioned that it usually takes close to a year to get off the medication that I had been on for two years; however, my body seemed to be just fine doing it in six months.

Do you think you there is hope for you?

Hope is the drive to change which can be easy for some and hard for others.

One day, I had an impression to make more desserts. Children (well, all people) especially tend to feel deprived when they are eating healthy or thinking of eating healthy. At this point, I was eating about 80% raw foods (uncooked), about 20% meat and cooked foods. When I was in an herb shop on June 26, 2013, I bought *Ani's Raw Food Desserts: 85 Easy, Delectable Sweets and Treats* by Ani Phyo. I also purchased *Faves* by Melissa Chappell from another store. With those books and others in hand, my children and I made all sorts of healthy desserts. I loved making the raw ice creams and especially loved Ani's Coconut Ice Kream, Strawberry-Coconut Cookies, Flax Bread, Liquid Chocolate and the cobblers in her book. My children, Tyler, Ashley, and Lana, made Melissa Chappell's No Bake No Bakes cookies all the time. We tried to recreate her Vanilla Macaroons that she sold in the local health food store, and I think we did an awesome job. She now has it in her dessert recipe book *Melt in your Mouth*. We also enjoyed making Melissa's Smoky Tomato Salsa and Energy Cereal. I made them all the time. We had a lot of fun with these and many other recipes, which really helped my children to adjust to this new way of eating.

As I went to classes, read books and read articles online, I told my kids what I was learning. I believe it helped them to understand why I was changing what we were eating. We found what foods we liked and what we did not like. My husband enjoyed the change because he loved eating vegetables.

He did not always agree with what I learned, although I knew in my heart what was true and what I was unsure of. When I learned about something I wasn't sure could be correct, I kept it in my mind and nearly always I would get a confirmation from another trusted source, like herbs for healing. For example, making raspberry tea when sick or during menstruation. One time I thought my daughter Lana might have strep throat, so I had her try the herbal or home remedy (which is 1 tablespoon raw honey, ¼ teaspoon cayenne [we used ⅛ teaspoon] and 2-3 cloves of fresh minced garlic, then mix it well and take a teaspoon every hour, having it sit in the back of your throat to drip down for the next 24 hours when awake). It was horrible and she had a hard time doing it perfectly. Despite that, her sore throat improved greatly by the next day. No need to go to the doctor for an antibiotic. I began to learn there was more than one way to heal and I was willing to try. If it did not work, then I had a doctor that I trusted.

I was eager to tell my friends what I was learning about food and nutrition, though I was a little cautious. Often people would think I was crazy. However, they wished they could be healthier. They would often say they could never do what I did: eat healthy. My friend Dana told me the same thing while we were living in her basement and again a year later in 2013 when we were visiting her and her husband. It was a few months after that I found out she had drastically changed her diet because she had been diagnosed with hyperthyroidism. Dana was so set on not being able to eat healthy because she was very busy while she was teaching high school during the day, teaching guitar at night, and working on her website in between. She loved the cookies people brought in at work, yet when faced with a disease, she did something about it.

You never know what seeds you plant will grow. I had more influence in helping others than I thought.

LEARNING ABOUT GAPS

While learning about health and nutrition, I was not only trying to heal myself but my son Wesley. During Christmas break 2012, his skin flared up incredibly bad when he got sick. I was happy to have a doctor I trusted, and we tried many things. In March of 2012, I was in a class about immunizations and asked the doctor, Jack Stockwell, about Wesley. The doctor advised me to read *GAPS* by Dr. Natasha Campbell-McBride about healing the gut. Dr. Stockwell felt most people needed to do this due to the type of foods we eat, which cause our bodies to be unable to digest the food properly. I purchased the *GAPS* book, yet I only read the first few pages and it sat on my shelf along with a few other books I wanted to eventually read. I did listen to Dr. Stockwell's radio show where he talked in detail about the gut and many other topics.

Have you had good intentions yet did not follow through?

During the next couple of years, (2012 - 2014) I was very consistent in cooking healthy whether it was vegetarian or eating Raw. During that time, my acid reflux and muscle tightening were not completely gone. I would feel great for a while and then it would come back. Every once in a while I would eat from the list of sensitive foods like dairy, onions, oranges, or even a piece of pizza to see how my body would do. Every time I tried, my acid reflux would return. As long as I kept off those foods, I felt fine. Would I ever be able to eat those foods again? I knew I should be able to eat bananas, oranges, grains, onions, plus many others from the list of sensitive foods I was avoiding.

During those two years, we tried different remedies and assistance from doctors to help my son heal his psoriasis. My husband Robert was told three times from friends about a doctor in a nearby town that we should go to for Wesley. He was my kind of holistic doctor, who used prescription drugs only when needed and started with the mildest. He worked with Wesley to reduce the candida in his body (candida - a yeast or fungal infection that can grow out of control in the digestive tract) and had him take homeopathic drops to aid his body in healing certain allergies to food and the environment. He made progress with his psoriasis, but it was never enough. Finally, I was prompted that the *GAPS* program was the answer. The doctor we were seeing at the time knew of the *GAPS* program and its intensity. He asked me several questions to help me understand what I was getting into. He wanted to try one more thing with my son. We tried it for the next three months without much improvement. The doctor said that he was not sure what else to do and put my son back into my hands. I told him that we were going to try the *GAPS* program. It was about August or September 2014 and Wesley was eighteen years old at this point.

During that time, I began to seriously read more of the *GAPS* book. Although I had not previously read much of the book, I had enough knowledge that by about October 2014 I told Wesley I really felt like this was the path to heal his psoriasis. I asked him to read the e-mail I sent him about the program and to pray about it. After doing so, he agreed to do the program and I asked him to pick a date to begin. Initially, he picked November 27, 2014, although, as Thanksgiving approached, we invited family over for pies the day after and so we moved our start date to November 28 (two days after Thanksgiving). You may wonder why we chose a date during the holidays. Well, there is never a good time to start - there is always a birthday party, a family gathering, lunch out with friends, a party at church or work, and of course, Christmas where there will be food we will miss out on. This date gave me two weeks to finish *GAPS* and understand what to do.

I decided Wesley needed someone he could talk to about how he was feeling physically and emotionally, plus someone to eat the same way as he did. I wasn't sure if this program could heal my acid reflux but I felt it would not hurt to try it so together we embarked on this road of healing.

With only two weeks to finish the book, understand the program, and with other responsibilities of a stay-at-home mom - my younger kids, my older kids, and other everyday duties - I knew I could not read the entire book in time, so I looked for assistance online. I watched Dr. Campbell-McBride's lecture she gave in London and other interviews with her. I also searched Amazon for another book to help me; I came across a gold mine which I recommend to my clients who are considering the *GAPS* program. It is *The Heal Your Gut Cookbook*. It was the best find. The two authors gave an explanation of the body and of the program. There is a chapter for each of the six stages of the introduction diet, along with recipes and helpful tips. I began to read the book online because I had no time to lose. I was told about an instructional video series on *GAPS* that was also amazing, taught by Vaughn Lawrence at *Spirit of Health* that I watched after we began the program.

I did not feel confident in the beginning although I felt as ready as I could be. I was a little nervous and not sure I could do the program. I worried about the restrictions, despite the fact I was already restricted in what I could eat. The unknown is always scary, and it seemed particularly daunting at the time. However, the day came and my hesitations disappeared immediately; we were on our way to healing. I was so excited.

I made some mistakes that first day by not having meat stocks and soups ready to go. I made three gallons of meat stock the day before, although I thought it needed to be cooked for 24 hours and so I did not have soups ready for breakfast the first day. I quickly learned that they only need to be cooked on the stove for two and a half to three hours or six hours in the crockpot. I knew we needed to eat lots of soup and realized that an adult needs a gallon of soup a day during the introduction diet in order to have enough energy. Yes, an entire *gallon*. It seems like a lot; although, you are not eating much during this time so that is what you need to feel full. My clients are often shocked when they hear that. I had a client tell me she was so weak and was not sure she could continue. I asked her if she was eating a gallon of soup each day. Her answer was no and she could see how that would make a difference.

Are you ready to begin your road to better health?

I did not understand that I was quite constipated and had been for as long as I could remember. It was so painful to go to the bathroom, and I thought I would never be able to go through birthing a baby. However, on the gut healing program, I experienced vast improvement.

I followed the program as designed by Dr. Campbell-McBride; I knew if I was going to go through all this trouble, then I would follow it 100%. I kept her book with me and re-read it often to make sure I was following it correctly (it is the "Bible" of the program). I added supplements - fish oils and enzymes as suggested. In two weeks, I noticed my fingernails were considerably stronger.

After a year on the program, my husband thought our son needed to do something different. I was not going to take him off the *GAPS* program; still, maybe I needed some help. So I decided to take him to see a *GAPS*-certified practitioner. The visit was helpful and her suggestions to add *Standard Process* supplements helped his healing. I also received a free visit with one of their nutritionists. It was a good visit and I decided to begin her supplement suggestions. It was expensive, and yet it propelled my body to further healing.

Sometimes we look back and wonder why we did not embark on a certain path sooner. The *GAPS* book was a wealth of information, yet it sat on my shelf for two years. After we noticed big changes, I asked myself why had I not read the book and put its treasures into practice earlier? The answer was that my son and I were not ready - not ready for what it would take to be involved or to be 100% committed. Wesley had told me he was not committed to staying off the foods he was sensitive to until then. It is hard to eat differently in social settings as a high school student and young adult. I completely understood. Later, he told me that we started it at the right time; he had felt his body was going to shut down. Another confirmation to being directed at the right time.

It was 2016 and I happily continued on the *GAPS* diet very secure in knowing that patience would be the key to healing, especially since the average time on the healing program was two years.

I was content to cook at home; nevertheless, when eating out I would actually get quite nervous. It was very scary and I would wonder why we had to eat out. Regardless, I told my husband or friends very cheerfully that I could make it work and I did. The key to survive eating out was to know the restaurants and not be afraid to ask questions. I asked a lot of questions so that I was eating what was on the approved list of foods. I often would create my own meal. I did not want to eat off the list because it would take my body a week or two to get back on track.

What health problem would you like to improve? Is it time for you to take action?

EMOTIONAL HEALING

Did you know that food is not the only key to healing?

In the beginning of my transformation, I did not truly understand that food was not the only way to heal. There was another piece of the healing puzzle that I neglected to dive into: emotional healing and forgiveness. When I began to add it to my physical healing, I saw longer-lasting improvements. Before delving into emotional healing, my acid reflux would return during stressful times and I was not sure that I was ready to go off the *GAPS* program even after being on the program for two years. I felt that if I was still experiencing acid reflux, it meant I was not yet healed. So I stayed on the program.

I fell into emotional healing because of a failed foot surgery recovery. The joint of my big toe was large with scar tissue, my foot was swollen, and it was beginning to be painful with every step. I finally decided to follow the suggestion from my naturopathic Dr. Paul Jensen to take action. I asked my chiropractor, Dr. Ashleigh Street to recommend a physical therapist which she did but I didn't follow through. When I went in for my next appointment I asked her again for the name the physical therapist she recommended last time. She suggested I try a foot zone therapist first. So I called Janine (the therapist she recommended) and explained my situation. Even though she was not sure she could help, I made an appointment. She asked if I wanted the foot zoning done with the emotional part and I agreed, not understanding what it was.

There are a lot of different emotional modalities like *EFT tapping* (I listened to a few webinars and even bought one. I felt it helped), *morning papers*, and *reiki* that can help. You can find one that works best for you.

After my first appointment, I found it helped my foot, so I made more appointments. I still don't understand how it works, although, it is along the lines of what is explained in the book *Emotion Code* by Bradley Nelson, clearing emotions stuck inside from the past and present. I also had Janine do *Innerwise and hypnosis* to help me through other trapped emotions and forgiveness of an abuse in my young adult years. Because of this type of emotional work I began to feel more confident and able to express my thoughts and feelings more to my husband and others, which helped improve our relationship. It was not easy for me to break old habits, nor easy for my husband, yet it was needed. Nevertheless, together we are better for it. **I am better for it!**

Since fear was released from my thoughts and feelings, I was no longer afraid to go off the *GAPS* program. On April 24, 2018, three and a half years after starting the program, I started the *coming off* portion of the program following Dr. Campbell-McBride's directions. You are supposed to come off the diet slower than you would with an elimination diet so you can really see if you are ready. I will still eat differently, but my variety will increase. Dr. Campbell-McBride says *GAPS* patients will never be able to eat as they did before.

Healing is not fast, it takes time to heal an injured body. I began my lifestyle change in March 2011 and at the time of writing this book (late 2018), eight years ago, which is a long time to be healing. I went to Janine, the foot zone therapist, for over a year before I began to see lasting shifts emotionally and in my foot. I rarely have acid reflux problems during stressful times now. Yet I was most likely sick longer than that and did not even know it. Our bodies are made so incredibly well they can take a lot of abuse and before showing signs of illness. Nevertheless, it can't do it forever; eventually there will be signs of illness. As you may have noticed in our day and age, children are getting what used to be considered adult diseases. Even old age illnesses, such as memory loss or other ailments, we see it as normal now. I don't believe it has to be that way.

As I stated in the beginning, patience is key to success. Take one step at a time as you are ready to, though don't take too long to make the necessary changes in order to see real healing happen.

In the next section, I will guide you through ten steps to improve your health. Make a plan to go through each step as you feel you are ready to. Don't get caught up on perfection before moving on. Each step is set up to build on the previous step. Some overlapping will occur and is expected to happen.

Many people find they can succeed on their own; however, some need additional support. I offer personal health coaching to assist in transformation, and as an Integrative Nutritional Health Coach, we will work together to help you succeed.

Section 2

10 Steps to a Healthier You!

Step One: Desire to Change

It may seem like a silly step, to begin with, but if you don't have the **desire** to make changes, they will not happen. Writing them down will help to cement them into your head and your heart.

In the spaces below, write down the reasons you are wanting to make a change.

Example: Health reasons such as fatigue, brain fog, memory, weight, skin, disease, to feel better, lose weight or your family's needs.

I am changing because:

____

____

____

____

____

> *TIP:* On the next page, make another copy and post it on your bathroom mirror. Seeing it each day will confirm your reasons for change and help to keep yourself on track to better health.

I AM CHANGING BECAUSE:

44

Step Two: Know Ingredients

Knowing which ingredients are unhealthy is the next step to change. It can be daunting. The list of ingredients to avoid can be quite large. As I mentioned earlier in my story, I was very distressed when I learned about and read about the ingredients on the foods I bought. My hope is that this will empower you to make better choices when at the store.

Foods you find in health food stores are not necessarily healthy. It is best to check labels there, too.

Below are examples what I avoided in the beginning, the list of "ingredients to avoid" and a list of "healthy ingredients". The following ingredients are unhealthy because they disrupt your body's system to function normally and increases the risk to disease. I have referenced websites where you can learn in more detail how they disrupt the body.

Use the ingredients to avoid as a guide. At this point in your transformation, it is **not necessary** to avoid all of them, just to **reduce** your exposure to the majority of them. As you learn about them and your body shifts, you will automatically cut more and more out as I did.

Examples of what I avoided in the beginning of my transformation:

Refined sugar: Refined cane sugar, high fructose corn syrup, corn syrup, and those ending with -ose plus artificial sweeteners. Instead, I bought products with organic cane sugar or syrup, invert sugar, tapioca syrup and malt syrup.

<u>MSG (Monosodium glutamate)</u>: I cut out as much of the MSG group as I could - the big ones are yeast extract, carrageenan, maltodextrin, soy anything, nitrates.

<u>Grains</u>: I tried to not buy anything enriched. 100% whole wheat.

<u>GMO</u>: I tried to keep away from GMO foods as I learned about them.

<u>Honey</u>: Bought raw honey when I learned that if the product contains 3% of something it does not have to be listed. Honey contains water and sugar.

<u>Oils</u>: hydrogenated, partially hydrogenated, vegetable and the rest as I learned about them.

<u>Preservatives</u>: the colors, sodium benzoate, sulfur

Here is the list of ingredients to avoid (not all-inclusive):

INGREDIENTS TO AVOID:

<u>Refined Sugar with its many names</u>: high fructose corn syrup; maize syrup, glucose syrup, fructose syrup, cane syrup, tapioca syrup, dahlia syrup, fruit fructose, crystalline fructose, corn syrup; anything that ends in "ose" - glucose, sucrose, dextrose, maltose, lactose, fructose; invert sugar, barley malt syrup, brown sugar, powdered sugar, glucose solids, artificial sweeteners: sucralose, aspartame, saccharin, cyclamate, agave (I've used it; however, it is debatable if it is a healthy sweetener even though it is low in glucose. See the "Notes" section).

<u>MSG</u>: glutamate, glutamic acid, monosodium glutamate, magnesium glutamate, natrium glutamate, gelatin, calcium caseinate, sodium caseinate, textured protein, hydrolyzed protein (anything hydrolyzed), yeast nutrient, yeast extract, yeast food, autolyzed yeast, vetsin,

ajinomoto, whey protein, soy protein, soy protein concentrate, soy protein isolate, whey protein, whey protein concentrate, whey protein isolate

<u>MSG: names of hidden msg</u>: carrageenan, bouillon and broth, stock, any "flavors" or "flavoring", maltodextrin, citric acid, citrate, anything "ultra-pasteurized", barley malt, pectin, protease, anything "enzyme modified", anything containing "enzymes", malt extract, soy sauce, soy sauce extract, anything "protein fortified", anything "fermented", seasonings

<u>Enriched and Fortified</u>: these are grains that have stripped the original parts of the food away to become white and added synthetic vitamins back into it. Example: enriched wheat flour and then listing vitamins.

<u>GMO</u>: genetically modified organisms: the main reasons for these foods is so that pesticides and herbicides can be used on them so that they can be sprayed and do not die. The chemical stays on the skin and is often digested.

<u>Honey</u>: traditional honey on the market is usually mixed with water and sugar. Like most packaged items, there is a percentage in which there is no need to label, usually 3%

<u>Oils</u>: vegetable, soybean, canola, hydrogenated - fully and partially; corn, shortening, cottonseed, grapeseed, margarine, safflower, and sunflower.

<u>Preservatives</u>: sodium benzoate, sodium nitrite, sodium sulfite, sulfur dioxide, propyl paraben, propyl paraben, bha and bht, yellow no. 5,

blue #1 and blue #2, red dye # 3 (also red #40), yellow #6 and yellow tartrazine, natural green color, natural flavors.

<u>Nuts and seeds</u>: Roasted, salted, and flavored.

Stay away from foods from China except for because they are grown in the mountains above the pollution.

INGREDIENTS THAT ARE HEALTHY:

<u>Sugar</u>: raw honey, stevia-green leaf powder is not refined and I like sweet leaf liquid and NuNaturals alcohol free stevia, dates, coconut sugar, coconut syrup, pure maple syrup, turbinado sugar, raw sugar, sorghum syrup.

<u>Grains</u>: 100% whole grains, grains in their whole form. For example: whole oat groats, whole buckwheat (which is really a seed), millet, quinoa, brown rice, and whole grain wheat.

<u>Oils</u>: avocado oil, extra virgin olive oil (best when cooking with using low to medium heat or no heat), coconut oil - unrefined or refined, lard (pork fat), tallow (beef fat), grass-fed butter, ghee made from grass-fed butter (it's better if homemade; it's nasty if purchased), sustainable palm oil, walnut oil (cook with low heat or no heat), sesame seed oil, peanut oil, pumpkin seed oil, pistachio oil, and hemp oils

<u>Raw nuts and seeds</u>: this means not roasted, salted, or flavored.

> **TIP:** Choose items that have fewer ingredients listed on the label.

Step Three: Vegetables and Fruits

As you begin to buy prepared foods with fewer ingredients, it is time to increase the amount of vegetables and fruit you consume. As you eat more produce each day you will notice that your cravings for unhealthy foods will begin to decrease. Why? It is because your body is getting the nutrients it needs. Unhealthy foods only fill you up, not feed you.

Do not worry about buying organic at this point; you need to add more vegetables and fruits to your daily consumption.

You can cook them or eat them raw. You may even begin to notice they have more flavor and taste better. This is one of the coolest things that happens when you begin to shift what you put into your mouth.

Write down two to three vegetables **and** fruits you will add in the next two weeks.

1.____

2.____

3.____

4.____

5.____

6.____

How are you going to prepare them? Soups? Salads? Raw? Cooked?

1. ____

2. ____

3. ____

4. ____

TIP: If you want to begin buying organic, you can begin with these four - cucumbers, lettuces, apples, and celery.

Step Four: Change Your Salt

Unrefined salt has over eighty essential minerals. Refined salt has no minerals, is bleached, and contains toxic ingredients such as ferrocyanide ammonium citrate and aluminum silicate. Plus, there is not enough iodine in iodized salt for all of our body's iodine needs.

As I mentioned in my story, I was greatly influenced by Dr. Brownstein's book "*Salt*". He says: "The first step to optimizing your health is to ensure the **adequate intake of healthy salt and water.** I firmly believe that salt and water form the foundation for any health treatment plan. It is *impossible* to achieve your optimal health in a dehydrated and salt-deficient state."

The American Heart Association and others have told us to limit our salt consumption. However, the reason we are consuming so much "bad" salt is because it is in all boxed, canned, and even fast foods, causing our bodies to be overloaded. As you begin to limit prepared foods you will be reducing your salt intake, therefore needing to add unrefined salt to your diet.

Look for colored salt or salt with specks of color. For example: Real Salt, Himalayan, Celtic or one that is not pure white.

Real Salt - for more salty flavor   Himalayan - for sweeter flavor
Celtic - very mild
Black - often used "raw" for mock eggs

TIP: Buy a small container of *Real Salt* and give it a try.

Step Five: Make Desserts

You are going to love this step! Yes, this step is to make desserts. Why? Because you need them. Dessert is so common in our culture and in all of our gatherings. When we think of being healthy, we think about all the delicious desserts we will be missing out on. Those desserts are the very things that cause us to lose sight of our goal.

So, I give you permission as a Health Coach to make all the desserts in the recipe section. Go to my website www.SuzyCooking.com for more desserts. Search online for other healthy desserts, being mindful of the ingredients. Some people have different visions of what makes a healthy ingredient.

Web Search: try searching "healthy desserts honey" - or put the type of dessert before honey, coconut sugar or other type of sweetener, paleo, gaps, etc.

TIP: Bring a dessert you enjoy to your next gathering for yourself only or to share.

Step Six: Reflection

Let's take time and think about these changes.

By taking time to ponder you will be able to understand how these changes are manifesting themselves in your life. It will help you to continue moving forward.

What three changes have been the most beneficial?

1. ____
2. ____
3. ____

What three changes do you feel you are consistent with?

1. ____
2. ____
3. ____

What three changes are you most worried about?

1. ____
2. ____
3. ____

Are you feeling different?

____

____

____

____

Write down why or how you are feeling different.

____

____

____

____

____

Next, take each worry and write down why you are worried. Is it something you need to deal with now or just let it pass as you keep on this road to better health?

1. ____

2. ____

3. ____

> **TIP:** During this next week, take one worry and decide what you will do about it and write it below. Do the same for the next two weeks.

Step Seven: Reduce Refined Sugar

If you have not done so already, begin to reduce the amount of refined sugar with all of its variations from your diet.

Refined sugars dull the senses. So watch your taste buds become alive in a way you never thought they could before. It is great to discover how much better everything tastes once you eliminate refined sugar from your diet. For example, you may have hated broccoli in the past, but now you find it tolerable.

However, I would not go cold turkey at this point in your transformation. Unless you have reason to do so, going cold turkey may cause you to quit your transformation (depending on what you are eating as of today). The common symptoms of withdrawal will be flu symptoms: aches, nausea, throwing up, headaches, chills, fatigue, etc.

As my friend and client began the *GAPS* program with her son, I soon discovered she had made no changes to the amount of sugar she was eating. Along with the detox she was doing at the start of the program, she was having sugar withdrawals (which can be similar to any heavy drug withdrawals). She felt like she was going to die. Finally, the fourth day brought recovery and by the end of the week, she felt changed for the better. She told me she looked at sugar in a different light. Considering what she ate especially when offered a "sugar" dessert. She was happy about the change.

> *TIP:* Don't try to eliminate refined sugar completely at this point in your transformation. You will naturally refuse to eat it as you continue on this path.

Step Eight: Water

Are you drinking water? If you find yourself thinking from time to time that you should be drinking more water, then chances are you are not drinking enough. Beverages like sodas, juices, coffee, or energy drinks do contain water; however, they also contain dehydrating agents.

Our bodies are made up of 60-75% water; the brain contains 85% water and it is not unusual to feel hungry, fatigue and headaches when your body is asking for water. Drinking too much water can cause mineral imbalances.

Finding the right amount depends on where you live, what you eat, and what you do. On average, men should consume thirteen cups and women nine cups. Increase your water intake if you live in a hot and humid area, if you live in altitudes above 8200 feet, if you are exercising (a lot), or for illness, infections, pregnancy/breastfeeding, or alcohol use. If you are eating fruits, leafy greens, or vegetables with water content, you may not need as much water.

Dr. F. Batmanghelidj said, "You're not sick; you're thirsty. Don't treat thirst with medication." In his book *Your Body's Many Cries for Water,* he also says that many ailments and symptoms are often improved or disappear when water is consumed. He says thirst should not be treated with medication and water is the foundation of life.

The type of water you drink makes a difference; however, at this point in your transition, I want you to look at how much water you drink and increase it if necessary.

Step Eight: Water

TIP: Begin your day with a glass of warm or room temperature water because cold water can aggravate any health condition you may have. You can add a little bit of lemon for a refreshing taste. Brush your teeth afterward because lemon juice is acidic on the teeth.

Step Nine: Meats and Fish

Switching to healthy meats and fish can be expensive. In the beginning of my transformation, I purchased meats that looked healthier than the standard meats available. I looked at labels like I was doing with boxed foods.

So, begin by purchasing meat from animals raised without hormones, antibiotics, MSG, nitrates, nitrites, and no added preservatives. Read the labels in the meat section and purchase the best quality you can find. Even if they are grain-fed, it is just fine at this point of your transformation.

For fish, buy wild caught. Since they are wild they are automatically without hormones and antibiotics.

If you don't find any better meats at your local store, try a health food grocery store in your area.

TIP: Don't be afraid to buy chicken (or other meats) with the skin and fat left on.

Step Ten: Clean Out Your Pantry

You may have already begun this step while learning about ingredients in step 2. Or you read the labels but pushing your canned and boxed foods to the back of your pantry. Knowing what is in your pantry and purging those foods is another thing. This can be a hard step because you will begin to feel badly about the money you spent on those items. It may feel like throwing away money. I felt that same pain; however, I pushed through it knowing that my health and that of my family was more important than the money I would be losing.

You should be able to return food that has not yet expired to the store as I did. I received store credit which I used for other food. Or, you can give them to a food bank or family members. When I asked my sisters if they wanted my food, I explained why I was getting rid of it and they took it.

Eliminating temptation gives you a boost toward a healthier you.

TIP: Put all unwanted foods into two boxes: One box to take back to the store and a second one to give away.

Congratulations! You have already come a long way already in *your* transformation to better health.

As you keep working on these steps, your transformation will become sustainable.

For more help, contact me for a free consultation.

E-mail: Suzanne@SuzyCooking.com
Website: www.SuzyCooking.com

Section 3

The Recipes

What do I eat now?

Here are some of the recipes I heavily relied on in the beginning of my transformation.

Recipes are used with permission Look in the notes section at the end of the book for web addresses where you can purchase the books.

For more recipes visit SuzyCooking.com. Feel free to use them as a guide to what you are eating **today**.

Contents:

Desserts
Beverages
Breakfast
Main Meals
Salads/Dressing
Sides

64

DESSERTS

Make these as often as you feel the desire for a sweet treat. OR if you are feeling like you can't keep eating this way.

Desserts can help get you through the sugar withdrawal period, as well as the emotional withdrawal from what we are accustomed to.

Alternatives for **agave**: raw honey, coconut nectar or real maple syrup

Apple and Blueberry Crumble

By: Sandra Ramcher from *Healing Foods Cooking for Celiacs, Colitis, Crohn's and IBS*

SCD (Specific Carbohydrate Diet) mentioned below in the recipe.

Serves 4

Filling

1.350 kg (2 lb 11 oz) Granny Smith apples - peeled, diced and cored

200 g (1 cup) frozen blueberries

1 tablespoon fresh orange juice

1 teaspoon lemon rind - grated

3 tablespoons honey

Crumble

100 g (1 cup) almond flour

60 g (¼ cup) cold butter

1 teaspoon honey

Preheat oven to 150C/300F

Butter a 20 cm/8-inch square baking tin

Place all of the ingredients, retaining 2 Tbs honey, in a medium size saucepan and cook covered on medium heat for 5 minutes. Remove lid and simmer on high for another 5 minutes. Drain the fruit of its juices in a sieve. Pour the juice back into the saucepan adding the remaining tablespoon of honey, and simmer until reduced down by half. Retain this syrup for later. Cool the fruit in refrigerator. Meanwhile, take the crumble by combining the almond flour, butter and honey in a food processor. Mix until chunky crumbs are formed. Place the crumble in the refrigerator for 10 minutes.

When the fruit has cooled down, place it into the prepared baking tin and top with the crumble.

Bake for 30 minutes or until crumble is golden brown. Serve warm, topped with a little cream or scd yogurt and the retained syrup.

Carrot Pineapple Cake

By Tiffany Perez from *At Tiffany's Table Eat Your Way to Health*

This recipe makes two cakes great for freezes no one for later. I have included the frosting mentioned following this recipe.

1 cup butter

2 ½ cups raw honey

6 eggs

1 16oz. Can crushed pineapple

5 cups shredded carrots

5 cups fresh-ground whole wheat flour

3 teaspoons cinnamon

2 teaspoons baking soda

2 teaspoons vanilla

1 teaspoon sea salt

½ teaspoon nutmeg

Pre-heat oven to 350°. Grease 5 loaf pans, or 2 rectangle 9x13 pans. In a mixing bowl cream honey and butter. Add eggs, pineapple and carrots. Mix in remaining ingredients. Pour into pans and bake 40 minutes or until toothpick inserted in middle comes out clean. Cool completely. Frost with Buttery Cream Cheese Frosting (page 124 of the author's book). This cake freezes very well.

Buttery Cream Cheese Frosting
By Tiffany Perez from *At Tiffany's Table Eat Your Way to Health*

One of my favorite frostings. Page numbers below are referenced in her book.

¼ cup butter (room temperature)
4 oz. cream cheese (room temperature)
¼ cup raw honey
⅛ teaspoon vanilla
1 teaspoon orange zest (optional)

Cream all ingredients together. Refrigerate any remaining frosting.

Serve on Cinnamon Rolls (page 45 of the author's book) or Orange Cake (page 85 of the author's book).

Chia Snowballs

By: Robyn Openshaw & Desiree Ward from *Healthy Holiday Favorites*

With 5 children home at the time the was made all the time. I used almond butter since I could not eat peanut butter. It is great with either.

Here's what the originator had to say about it: " This recipe couldn't be any easier, and the snowballs present beautifully. Give people a healthful."

1 cup peanut butter or almond butter (preferable natural, without added sugar)
½ cup honey (raw)
½ cup brown rice syrup (found at health food stores)
4-5 cups brown rice cereal (found at health food stores)
3 tablespoons chia seeds
optional: 1 cup finely shredded coconut

Mix all ingredients together except for the coconut. Roll the mixture into balls and then roll in the coconut. Or, if omitting the coconut, press mixture into an 8x8 inch pan and refrigerate for 1 hour to let them set up. Store cookies in the refrigerator.

Note: Chia seeds are a power food. Packed with nutrition, they contain 19-23 percent protein. Two ounces of chia seeds will give you more Omega-3 than 1 ¾ pounds of salmon. Chia also has three times more flavonal (to fight cancer) than blueberries.

Effortless Peanut Butter Cookies
By: Robyn Openshaw & Desiree Ward from *Healthy Holiday Favorites*

These are so easy and very delicious. I have a raw honey version on my website.

Here is what the originator has to say about it: "....If you are wondering what to take for the holidays to a loved one or a friend that has a gluten intolerance, this would be the perfect gift."

Makes 1 dozen

1 cup chunky, all-natural peanut butter
1 cup coconut sugar
1 egg (organic, free-range)
1 teaspoon vanilla
conditional: ¼ teaspoon sea salt (only if the peanut butter has no added salt!)

Preheat the oven to 350°. Mix the egg and coconut sugar (and salt, if using) in a mixing bowl on medium speed until creamy. Add the peanut butter and vanilla until smooth.

For uniform cookies, use a cookie scoop to drop the dough onto a cookie sheet, then flatten them with a fork in a criss-cross pattern. Bake for 8-12 minutes.

Variation: Effortless Peanut Butter Oatmeal Cookies
Pulse ½ cup of rolled oats in a blender to break them up a bit. Follow the recipe above, adding the oats to the dough.

No Bake No Bakes
By Melissa Chappell from *Faves*

Melissa made No Bake Cookies from her childhood into a healthier version. She gives you permission to eat it right out of the bowl. Delicious they are!

makes 15 - 20 cookies

4 cups rolled oatmeal
1/2 cup almond butter
1/2 cup coconut oil
1 tablespoon vanilla
6 T cocoa powder
3/4 - 1 cup agave
3/4 teaspoon salt

Mix by hand in a bowl. Drop by spoonfuls on wax paper lined cookie sheet. Put in freezer until hardened. Eat and enjoy. For a holiday version I like to add 2-3 drops of cinnamon essential oil to the mix.

Pecan Caramel Toffees

By: Sandra Ramcher from *Healing Foods Cooking for Celiacs, Colitis, Crohn's and IBS*

Here's what the originator had to say about it: "Warning Beware of the Pecan Toffees. They are addictive."

She is right!! We made these with almond butter and they were delicious.

Makes about 40
300 g (1 cup) honey
240 g. (1 cup) nut butter*
2 tablespoons butter
80 g (¾ cup) pecans - chopped

Place the honey into a medium sized pot and bring to boil. The honey will froth up. Keep boiling for about 8 minutes. Turn off the heat, add the nut butter, butter, and chopped pecans. Remove the pot from the heat and let cool for about 10 minutes. Place about 1 teaspoon of the toffee into individual candy cups and refrigerate. Eat at room temperature.

*use cashew butter, peanut butter or macadamia butter. Any nut butter is fine, as long as it does not contain any additives like sugar.

Pumpkin Pie
By: Suzanne Stevens

1 pie

Ingredients
3/4 cup raw honey
1 1/2 teaspoons ground cinnamon
1 teaspoon ground cloves
3/4 teaspoon ground allspice
1/2 teaspoon ground ginger
1/2 teaspoon salt
1/2 teaspoon vanilla
4 large eggs
2 cups pureed pumpkin
1/2 cup raw milk, coconut milk or nut milk

Directions:
1. Pre-heat oven to 425° .
2. Mix all ingredients together.
3. Bake 15 minutes
4. Turn oven temperature to 350° for 45-60 minutes, until knife comes out clean.

Pie Crust
By: Suzanne Stevens

Yield: makes 1 deep dish 10" pie shell.

Ingredients:

1 1/2 cups whole wheat flour - plain flour, not self-rising.

1/2 teaspoon salt (optional)

3 tablespoons coconut oil

1/3 cup COLD butter

1/4 cup cold water

Directions:

1. Mix the flour, sugar and butter first. About 15 seconds in a food processor is by far the best way, since it is fast and the ingredients don't warm up much. Don't make it too smooth or uniform. Little pea sized granules makes a flaky crust. Don't over mix.

2.Then sprinkle in the water, just enough water to make it hold together; a good dough consistency.

3. Chill dough for half an hour or more wrapped in plastic or a ziplock bag. If not then roll out the dough or press it into the pie plate.

4. Fill and bake pie according to pie directions.

Shortbread Cookies

By Tiffany Perez from *At Tiffany's Table Eat Your Way to Health*

Kids will ask for more. Be careful not to over cook or they will be dry. No need to worry though they will still be devoured.

1 stick butter
¼ cup raw honey
1 cup fresh-ground whole wheat or spelt flour

Pre-heat oven to 350°. In a mixing bowl cream butter and honey. Add flour, mix just until blended. Pat with wet hands into an un-greased square or round baking dish. Bake 15-20 minutes until edges browned and it is cooked through. Score lightly into wedges, let cool in the pan.

When cooled run knife around edges, carefully dump out onto the counter. Turn over and cut according to the score lines. This should be crisp and crunchy once it has cooled.

*Make sure this is completely cooled before trying to get it out of the pan, or it will just fall apart. Once it has cooled completely it should slide right out when turned over.

Tiffany's Brownies

By Tiffany Perez from *At Tiffany's Table Eat Your Way to Health*

1 stick plus 2 tbsp butter

8 tbsp cocoa powder, or carob powder, or 50% cocoa and 50% carob powder

1 ¼ cups raw honey

2 teaspoons vanilla

3 eggs (best at room temperature)

¼ cup plain yogurt

1 cup fresh-ground whole wheat or spelt flour

Pre-heat oven to 350°. In a small saucepan on low heat melt butter and cocoa powder together, let cool flighty. Cream honey, vanilla, eggs and yogurt in a mixing bowl. Add cocoa mixture to honey mixture. Stir in flour, just until blended. Pour into a greased, square baking dish. Bake 45 minutes.

Yellow Cake

By Lauren Hoover-West from recipe book *NO WHEAT, NO DAIRY, NO PROBLEM!* https://nowheatnodairynoproblem.com/cookbook-orders/

Here's what the originator had to say about it: "A moist and delicious cake that can be transformed into many variations…. Makes the perfect children's birthday cake!"

I have included the Chocolate Ganache Frosting she mentions in this recipe directly after it. I used coconut oil to grease the pans.

Yields: 1 (9x13) cake or two 8 inch round cakes

3 ½ cups oat flour

2 teaspoons baking soda

2 teaspoons baking powder

1 teaspoon sea salt, fine

¼ cup grapeseed oil

2/3 cup coconut nectar or real maple syrup

2 cups coconut milk or unsweetened almond milk*

2 teaspoons apple cider vinegar

1 tablespoon real vanilla extract or 2 vanilla beans

Preheat oven to 350°. Oil pan with vegan Earth Balance or grapeseed oil, then dust with oat flour and tap out any excess. Sift all dry ingredients into the bowl of an electric stand mixer or a bowl and use an electric hand mixer. Measure out all liquid ingredients and add to dry ingredients. If using vanilla beans, cut in half lengthwise and scrape out seeds with the back of a knife. Whisk the vanilla bean seeds into the wet ingredients. Put vanilla pod into a bag of sucanat or maple sugar to flavor. Place paddle attachment onto mixer and mix on low speed just until incorporated. Stop mixer and scrape down sides and bottom of the bowl, mix briefly just until combined over mixing will make the cake tough. Pour batter into cake pan and bake on the middle rack of oven for 40 minutes. Insert a toothpick in the middle of the cake and it is done when it comes out clean. If it does not come out clean continue baking approximately 5 more minutes or until toothpick comes out clean. Cool on a wire rack until completely cool. Remove from round pans. You can keep it in the 9x13 pan. Frost with "Buttercream" or Chocolate Ganache (see index). This unfrosted cake can be double wrapped in plastic and then put into a freezer plastic zip bag and frozen for up to one month.

*unsweetened rice or soy milk may be substituted

Chocolate Ganache

By Lauren Hoover-West from recipe book *NO WHEAT, NO DAIRY, NO PROBLEM!* https://nowheatnodairynoproblem.com/cookbook-orders/

Here's what the originator had to say about it: "This is the most versatile sauce. It can be used for an ice "cream" topping, dessert sauce, frosting and truffles. It is thick and fudgy when it is cold and thin and syrupy when it is warm. What's not to like about that Absolutely nothing! Shh, it's great to just scoop out of the jar when it's cold for that sweet tooth fix! Ganache is simply equal parts of chocolate and cream, but we will use coconut milk instead of cream."

Yields: 3 cups-enough to frost one 9x12 cake or double layer 8 inch round cake or 3 dozen cupcakes
12 ounces dark chocolate (Valrhona, Callebaut,
Dagoba, Green and Blacks) or chocolate chips**
1 ½ cups regular coconut milk (not light)
½ cup Valrhona cocoa powder, optional but recommended!

*For sweeter frosting you can add ¼ cup coconut nectar or real maple syrup to the coconut milk, optional

Place chocolate in a metal or glass bowl and set aside. Put coconut milk in a saucepot and bring to a boil, pour over chopped chocolate. See note for sweeter frosting above-if using chocolate chips it will be sweet enough. Let it sit for 1-2 minutes and then stir with a silicone spatula until smooth and well mixed.

For a shiny glaze over cake: pour directly over cake and let it set at room temperature for a few hours-do not refrigerate. Best when the cake is in a pan. If you are doing it over a round cake on a stand, pour half over it and let it set and then pour the other half so it doesn't all run to bottom of the cake onto the stand and not on your cake! For a fluffy frosting: Chill the Ganache in the refrigerator until it is completely set and thick like fudge. Put into an electric stand mixer, fitted with the paddle attachment, and mix on medium-high speed until it is fluffy. For a really deep, dark chocolate flavor, add ½ cup Valrhona cocoa powder, and mix on low speed until smooth and completely incorporated. For sweeter frosting you can add ¼ cup coconut nectar or real maple syrup to the coconut milk, optional. The amount of coconut nectar or real maple syrup will depend on the bitterness of the chocolate that is used. Spread onto the cake and leave at room temperature or refrigerate to use later.

For chocolate sauce or topping: use warm. Let Ganache cool to room temperature and then store it in a glass jar or container with a lid in the refrigerator. Never put warm or hot food directly into any plastic as it releases toxins that can be absorbed into your food. Spoon out the amount you need and heat on low over stove, stirring constantly so it does not burn or microwave in 10 second intervals, stirring in between-it can burn in the microwave too.

Wonderful over ice "cream" or alongside cake or over fresh fruit or berries. See the ice "cream" soda recipe too. You can put this into a fondue pot and keep it warm and serve a platter of fruit and cut up cake cubes to dip in the chocolate fondue (see index).

**Be sure the chocolate chips are dairy free

BEVERAGES

Almond Milk/Hazelnut Milk

By Lauren Hoover-West from recipe book *NO WHEAT, NO DAIRY, NO PROBLEM!* https://nowheatnodairynoproblem.com/cookbook-orders/

This a great recipe for those needing to be diary free. Make with or without the sweetener. Lauren Hoover-West says that the milk will last one week in the fridge. I have found it depends on how cold your fridge is. So best to check it in three days.

2 1/2 cups raw organic almonds or hazelnuts

6 cups filtered water

1 teaspoon real vanilla extract, optional

coconut nectar or real maple syrup, optional

If you are using almonds, place them in a glass or plastic container and cover with filtered water and refrigerate for 12 hours to make them more digestible. Drain and rinse. Hazelnuts do not need to be soaked because they do not have an enzyme inhibitor.

Place nuts and filtered water into blender. Pulse on low until the water turns white, and nuts are small chunks. If you over mix the nuts and they are too fine, the milk will not be smooth.

Add 1 teaspoon vanilla extract and coconut nectar or real maple syrup to taste if desired. Drain through fine trainer or cheesecloth and squeeze out extra liquid. Save nuts for hummus or sprinkle on cereal or salad.

The milk will keep in the refrigerator for 1 week. Place a sticker with a best. before date on the container. I like to keep it in a glass pitcher or glass mason jar. You can freeze it- just shake it as it may separate when defrosted.

Use in place of milk in any recipe, eat with cereal or make a smoothie by adding fruit!

Holiday Green Smoothie
{Raw Recipe}

By: Robyn Openshaw & Desiree Ward from *Healthy Holiday Favorites*

I didn't even know what a persimmon was at the time. I did find them and we tried this green smoothie out. I replace it with the raw milk or yogurt since I was not familiar with kefir. Any type of milk or milk replacement will do.

Here is what the originator has to say about it: "Forget the power struggle over getting your kids to eat their greens. Give them this smoothie and they will be begging for more! High in vitamin C, this smoothie will help you fight off winter colds. "

 4 persimmons
1-2 frozen bananas
2 cups almond milk
½ cup plain kefir
½ avocado
2 cups spinach
2 cups kale
1 tablespoon chia seeds
optional: 1-3 teaspoons. Agave (raw, organic)

Blend all ingredients in a high-powered blender for about 1-2 min.

Lemon Water
By: Suzanne Stevens

After reading *The pH Miracle* book from Robert O. and Shelley Redford Young. I would drink this first thing in the morning. Also throughout the day.

Ingredients:
1 cup room temperature or warm water
A squeeze or two of fresh lemon juice to taste

Directions:
Combine and enjoy.

Notes:
Lemon is alkaline for the body but acidic for your teeth. Be sure to brush.

Strawberry Mint Smoothie
By Melissa Chappell from *Faves*

Serves 2

The mint flavor of this smoothie is very addicting. I did not have wintergreen essential oil on hand so I used peppermint essential oil and the taste reminds me of Christmas. I recommend using the either essential oil because that is what makes this drink so awesome.
Here is what the originator has to say about it "I use this smoothie when teaching my "Beginning Fresh" workshops. It works well as an introduction to putting green things into one's smoothies because mint is a familiar flavor with the sweet tang of strawberries. Be sure to use organic berries, as strawberries are on the "dirty dozen" list of the most pesticide-laden foods, when conventionally grown."

3 cups frozen strawberries

¼ cup water

1 teaspoon honey

1 Red Delicious apple

2 tablespoons fresh mint

¼ cup almonds

1 drop wintergreen essential oil (optional)

Without peeling or seeding your apple, coarsely chop it and add it to your blender. Add the rest of the ingredients and blend until smooth. Serve immediately with a sprig of mint on top and a couple slices of fresh strawberries if you've got them.

Watermelon Drink
By: Ashley Stevens

My daughter Ashley created this drink one day when we had a lot of watermelon leftover.

Ingredients:
1 watermelon
1 - 1 ½ cups strawberries fresh or frozen
1 medium or large lemon juiced

Directions:
1. Rough cut enough watermelon to fill the blender leaving room for the strawberries.
2. Put watermelon, strawberries and fresh lemon juice in the blender.
3. Blend till done. You may need to still it around or use a tamper stick to get the blender going.
4. Enjoy.

Notes:
1. Add more strawberries for a creamier version.
2. Frozen strawberries will make it a cooler drink.

The next four smoothies are by Robyn Openshaw from *The Green Smoothies Diet*

Below are a few of her tips:

For beginners and kids, try using fewer greens and more fruit in the beginning. Then transition to using 50% greens and 50% fruits and build from there as your taste shifts.

The following recipes will yields six pints and are most easily made in a 96-ounce container. If you don't have one just cut the recipes in half.

Smoothies can last up to 24 hours in the fridge before they begin to lose their nutritional benefit. So for a single person make the large batch or one of her recipes, drink one quart that day, put a quart in the fridge for the next day and freeze the last quart for the third day. Shake well before drinking.

I (Suzanne Stevens) found this will save you time each day as you begin to get use to cooking more at home. I tested these smoothies on beginners and they enjoyed each of them. The greens in these recipes may shock you, nevertheless, this is a great way to be introduced to new vegetables.

Three of the recipes use frozen bananas. Plan ahead, peel and break banana into chunks and freeze. One recipe uses fresh frozen orange juice. Juice an orange into ice cube tray to freeze.

Cabbage Cool-Aid
By: Robyn Openshaw from *The Green Smoothies Diet*

Honey works well in this recipe.

Makes 6 pints

2 3/4 cups water/ice
Green cabbage, added until mixture reaches 6-cup line (yu choy or
bok choy works, too)
4 cups frozen mixed berries
2 large tart apples
¼ cup raw, organic agave

Blend first 2 ingredients until smooth. Add fruit and agave and blend
until smooth. Serve immediately for best results, or refrigerate up to
24 hours in glass jars and shake well before serving.

Dandelion Delight

By: Robyn Openshaw from *The Green Smoothies Diet*

Makes 6 pints

4 cups dandelion greens, coarsely chopped (wild/unsprayed, or found in health food stores)

½ teaspoon Stevia

¼ cup frozen orange juice (freshly squeezed adn frozen in ice cube trays -- 2 large ice cubes is ¼ cup)

Spinach, added and blended to the 6-cup line

2 oranges

2 bananas, frozen in chunks

¼ whole lemon

Frozen berries added until container is very full

Blend first 4 ingredients until smooth. Add fruit and blend again until smooth. Serve immediately for best results, or refrigerate up to 24 hours in glass jars and shake well before serving.

Mango Meltaway

By: Robyn Openshaw from *The Green Smoothies Diet*

The stevia in this recipe is liquid.

Makes 6 pints

2 3/4 cups water/ice
2 stalks celery, chopped in fourths
Spinach, added until mixture reaches 6-cup line
½ cup cashews
½ teaspoon vanilla
½ teaspoon stevia
2 large mangoes, peeled and cut away from the pot
2 bananas, frozen in chunks
2 cups frozen blueberries
½ cup plain, nonfat yogurt or kefir

Blend first 4 ingredients until smooth, then add remaining ingredients and blend again until very smooth. Serve immediately for best results, or refrigerate up to 24 hours in glass jars and shake well before serving.

Pear Date Puree
By: Robyn Openshaw from *The Green Smoothies Diet*

Makes 6 pints

2 3/4 cups water/ice

4 cups rainbow chard

Spinach, added until mixture reaches 6-cup line

¼ whole lemon

1 inch fresh ginger, peeled

6 large dates, or ½ chopped dates (rinsed)

3 large D'Anjou pears

3 cups frozen mixed berries

If possible soak dates in water for 30 minutes. Blend first 6 ingredients until smooth. Add pears and berries and blend again until smooth. Serve immediately for best results, or refrigerate up to 24 hours in glass jars and shake well before serving.

BREAKFAST

This one of the hardest meals to know what to make. Try these for a tasty change.

Energy Cereal
By Melissa Chappell from *Faves*

Here is what the originator has to say about it "I love to eat and I am hungry often. I'd love to eat constantly, but I'm a busy girl and sometimes I eat in the morning and then don't get a chance to eat again until late afternoon. On those days, I choose this cereal for breakfast. It fills me up and sustains me for hours. I like to add a little organic plain yogurt for creaminess and sometimes I'll also add other things like dates or sesame seeds. Don't be afraid to substitute other ingredients. For example, you might try golden raisins and almonds, or chopped, dried apricots and hazelnuts in place of the cranberries and pecans. Writing this is making me hungry. I'm gonna go make some right now."

Makes enough for about 15 portions.
10 cups rolled oats (long cooking)
1 cup dried cranberries (fruit juice sweetened, not sugar sweetened, available at any health food store)
1 cup pumpkin seeds
1 cup sunflower seeds
1-2 cups shredded coconut (unsweetened, available at any health food store)
½ cup flax seeds
1-2 cups almonds, pecans or macadamia nuts
Use oats as a base and add any or all of the rest of the ingredients or pick your own favorite dried fruits, nuts and seeds. Mix together and store in an airtight container and keep in your cupboard or pantry. To eat, soak about ⅔ cup of the dry cereal with water, milk, yogurt, or nut milk. Add frozen berries, and/or bananas or other fresh fruit, and honey, agave or maple syrup to taste for 5-10 minutes. You may also soak the cereal overnight in the fridge.

Pancakes

By: Sandra Ramcher from *Healing Foods Cooking for Celiacs, Colitis, Crohn's and IBS*

I bought her previous recipe book after the electrodermal test showed I sensitivity to grains. I had to learn how to cook and eat.

SCD (Specific Carbohydrate Diet) mentioned below in the recipe. These pancakes are a great alternative to wheat pancakes.

Serves 4

3 eggs
1 tablespoon scd yogurt
1 tablespoon honey
100 g (1 cup) almond flour
½ teaspoon baking soda

Beat eggs, yogurt, and honey until light and fluffy. Add almond flour and baking soda and stir until well combined. Heat a non-stick pan with a little oil. Pour in ⅓ cup of batter into the pan and fry until bubbles appear and the underside is golden brown. Flip and brown the other side. Serve warm with scd yogurt and our stewed apples or butter honey.

Pumpkin Oatmeal Waffles or Pancakes

By: Robyn Openshaw & Desiree Ward from *Healthy Holiday Favorites*

I did not understand what kefir was at the time I purchased this book so I used yogurt. This is a different twist to traditional pancakes. My family loves it best with strawberry sauce.

Here is what the originator has to say about it "These are Robyn's favorite "weekend" breakfast—pumpkin pie in the form of waffles!"

Serves 8

2 cups whole-wheat flour (finely ground, soft white wheat preferable)

2 cups regular rolled oats

1 (30 oz.) can pumpkin

¼ cup coconut oil (liquid)

3 tablespoons Sucanat

2 teaspoons cinnamon

1 teaspoon nutmeg

1 teaspoon sea salt

1 ½ teaspoons baking powder (no aluminum) -- reduce by ½ tsp. if you soaked grains overnight

1 cup plain yogurt or kefir

2 ½ cups water

2 teaspoons vanilla

3 eggs (organic, free-range)

Mix the rolled oats in your high-powered blender to break them down to a coarse meal. Mix the whole-wheat flour, oats, yogurt, and water together, then cover and let sit overnight. In the morning, add the remaining ingredients and mix by hand, but don't overmix. Batter is dense, and baking time usually must be longer than waffle timer indicates.

Top with quick applesauce for Waffles/Pancakes (page 46 of the author's book), Hot Caramel Apple Topping (page 22 of the author's book) or maple syrup.

Strawberry Syrup
By: Suzanne Stevens

I put a pot on the stove before I begin making pancakes and waffles so that they ready. Use whatever frozen fruit you have. Have a fruit syrup will cut down on the amount if any maple syrup you use.

Ingredients:
2 cups frozen strawberries

Directions:
1.   Put strawberries in a covered pot on medium.
2.   Stirring occasionally mashing berries as they soften.
3.   Uncover when juices are released.
4.   When berries are soft mash with your spoon or a masher to break them apart.

Serve over pancakes, waffles or on top of yogurt.

Notes:
Add honey or other sweetener if desired.

Good Morning Breakfast Bars

By: Sandra Ramcher from *Healing Foods Cooking for Celiacs, Colitis, Crohn's and IBS*

Use vanilla in place of vanilla essence. Once hard I cut a bar into pieces add it to my yogurt along with a berry sauce. I found it is very sweet if it gets too soft. If it too sweet for you make it with ¾ cup of honey.

300 g (1 cup) honey

35 g (⅓ cup) butter
160 g (1 cup) mixed nuts
60 g (1 cup) shredded coconut
90 g (½ cup) pitted dates - chopped
90 g (½ cup) pitted prunes- chopped
90 g (½ cup) pitted apricots - chopped
1 teaspoon vanilla essence

Preheat oven oven to 180C/360F.
Line a 20 cm (8 inch) square cake tin with baking paper.
Heat honey and butter in a saucepan, stir until butter has melted and is well combined with the honey. Turn off the heat and add all the other ingredients. Mix well and pour into the prepared cake tin. Bake for 30 minutes. Cool in refrigerator until set. Cut into bars and store between baking paper in an airtight container in refrigerator.
These bars need to be eaten straight from the refrigerator as they soften too much with warmer temperatures.

MAIN MEALS

20-minute Alkaline Stir Fry

By: Robert O. and Shelley Redford Young from *The pH Miracle*

1 package buckwheat soba noodles

½ package extra-firm tofu, cubed

Bragg Liquid Aminos, to taste

Vegetable broth, as needed

1 red bell pepper, chopped

1 onion, chopped

1 head broccoli, cut into florets, and/or

1 bunch asparagus, cut into 1-inch lengths

Olive oil

Raw, unhulled sesame seeds

Garlic

Stir-fry spice combination and/or ginger

Break noodles into fourths, prepare according to package directions, and drain. While the noodles are cooking, sauté tofu, in a large pan, in a little Bragg's and vegetable broth for about 5 minutes. Remove from pan and set aside. Sauté veggies for about 5 minutes in more Bragg's and broth. Add tofu and noodles. Sprinkle with olive oil, sesame seeds, garlic, and spices and stir gently.

Broccoli Creamed Soup

By: Robert O. and Shelley Redford Young from *The pH Miracle*

I have made this without the lecithin powder and it is still a yummy thick soup.

Serves 6

4 cups chopped broccoli
1 medium to large turnip, cut
2 cups pure water
½ cup celery, chopped
½ teaspoon Real Salt
1 chopped onion
Dash white pepper
2 tablespoons oil
½ quart vegetable broth
1 heaping teaspoon lecithin powder

Carefully sauté celery and onion in oil. Add broth, 1 cup water, and broccoli. Cook over medium heat until broccoli is tender-crisp. Meanwhile, steam turnip until hot, but not very soft. Allow to cool slightly and puree with enough water to ge a thick, smooth consistency. Add lecithin to blender and continue for a fe seconds to mic. Add puree to soup and season. Cook for a few minutes to thicken.

Chicken Stir-Fry

By: Suzanne Stevens

Not knowing what to eat I made this a lot. Use any veggies you have on hand or desire to consume.

Ingredients:

1-2 tablespoons coconut oil or olive oil or avocado oil

1 chicken breast cut into small pieces

1 onion chopped or sliced

2-3 peeled carrots and chopped or sliced

2 celery stalks sliced

½ - 1 whole broccoli florets

1 handful snow peas

¼ - ½ chopped cabbage

2-3 garlic

Directions:

1. Have all veggies and chicken chopped and ready to cook.

2. Heat oil in large cooking pan.

3. Lightly cook chicken on both sides.

4. Add the onion, carrots, celery and cook till onions begin to soften.

5. Then add the broccoli, snow peas, cabbage and garlic.

6. Cook to desired softness.

7. Top over brown rice.

Roasted Butternut/Celery Soup with Caramelized Onions
By: Robert O. and Shelley Redford Young from *The pH Miracle*

I made this without roasting the squash, celery, and onion. Tastes just as delicious.

Here is what the originator has to say about it: "This soup is a satisfying soup for chilly autumn and winter days. It is also delicious made with pumpkin and makes a great breakfast, lunch, dinner, or snack."

Serves 6-8
2 butternut squash
3 celery stalks, cut in big chunks
1 onion, peeled and chopped to big chunks
1 onion, peeled and sliced into this rings for garnish
2 tablespoons olive or Udo's oil
3-4 cups veggie stock (I use Pacific Foods of Oregon brand)
Cinnamon and nutmeg or salt and pepper, to taste

Cut squash in half and remove seeds. Lightly oil the cut side of the squash and chunks of celery and onion. Place squash cut side down and celery and onion chunks on an oiled cookie sheet and roast in a 400 degree oven for about 45 minutes or until tender and lightly browned. Scoop out soft squash from the skins.
Puree the roasted vegetables in a blender or food processor with some of the stock. If you'd like a smoother texture, pass the soup through a strainer into a clean pot. Add the rest of the stock, season to taste, and keep warm.
To make the onions ring garnish, fry the onion in oil for 10 minutes until brown and somewhat crisp. Top soup and serve immediately.

Shelley's Super Tortillas
By: Robert O. and Shelley Redford Young from *The pH Miracle*

Serves 6-8

4 cups flour (use any mix of flours you like, such as whole wheat, unbleached white, or spelt)
2 teaspoons Real Salt
4 teaspoons Seasoning of your choice (I use Spice Hunter's Mexican and California Pizza)
2 tablespoons dried onions
12 sun-dried tomatoes (packed in olive oil)
2 teaspoons Garlic powder
2-4 leaves fresh basil
1 ½ cups coconut milk or water
2 tablespoons olive oil

Mix all ingredients in a food processor with a dough S-blade. Use the pulse-chop action to prevent overheating the motor. When the dough forms into a one big ball, turn out onto a floured flat surface and break off balls and roll them out to about ⅛- to ¼-inch thickness. Transfer to an electric pan that has been lightly oiled and heat on both sides until you see a few air pockets rise. Take off the burner and let cool, then wrap in an airtight bag and keep in the fridge or freezer. Do not overcook, unless you want a crisped tortilla to use with dips or soups. Or you can decrease the milk or water and add fresh vegetable juices instead, such as spinach, parsley, or carrot.

Swedish Meatballs

By Lauren Hoover-West from recipe book *NO WHEAT, NO DAIRY, NO PROBLEM!* https://nowheatnodairynoproblem.com/cookbook-orders/

Here is what the originator has to say about it: "Whether you are 6 or 96, you will love these tender and flavorful little meatballs covered in gravy. Serve them over mashed potatoes, rice pasta noodles or rice. They make great leftovers and reheat very well. "

Yields: 24 meatballs, serves 4

1 lg. organic egg

1/ cup almond milk

¼ cup grated yellow or white onion

1 clove garlic, grated

½ teaspoon freshly grated whole nutmeg

½ teaspoon ground allspice

¼ teaspoon ground cardamom

1 teaspoon sea salt or kosher salt

Freshly ground pepper to taste

1 pound ground turkey (not all white meat)*

1 tablespoon olive oil

1 tablespoon grapeseed oil

2 Tablespoons oat flour

2 cups organic chicken stock or broth*64

2 teaspoons fresh dill or 2 Tablespoons fresh parsley, chopped finely

Preheat oven to 350°. Mix first 9 ingredients in an electric mixer with the paddle attachment until combined. Add ground turkey and mix until well combined. With a 2 ounce ice cream scooper, scoop meat mixture onto a 12 inch ovenproof or stainless steel or cast iron frying pan. For larger batches, use a baking sheet lined with parchment. Be sure the meatballs have just enough space between them so they don't touch. Bake on middle rack of the oven for 30 minutes. With a pot holder, remove from oven and add oil then flour to center of pan mixing until combined-If you baked the meatballs on a baking sheet, do this in a separate sauté pan. Pour chicken stock/broth into pan and whisk to make gravy. Add meatballs to gravy if they are on a baking sheet. Return to the oven and bake for 30 more minutes. Remove and sprinkle with dill or parsley and serve immediately.

*You can substitute ground beef or lamb for turkey and use beef stock/broth.

Sweet Potato Curry

By: Robyn Openshaw & Desiree Ward from *Healthy Holiday Favorites*

So easy to make and delicious this soon became our favorite curry. Here is what the originator has to say about it "To make this curry more traditional, use fish sauce -- but you can also substitute an equal amount of Nama Shoya."

Serves 4-5

1 medium carrot, peeled and cut into chunks

1 small sweet potato, cut inch 1" cubes

1 onion, cut lengthwise

½ red pepper, seeded and cut lengthwise in strips

1 ½ - 2 tablespoons yellow curry paste

1 can (13.5 oz) coconut milk

⅓ cup water

4 teaspoons Fish sauce or Nama Shoya (organic, unpasteurized soy sauce found at health food stores and online)

3 ½ teaspoons Sucanat

2 teaspoons tamarind juice

Heat the olive oil in a large saucepan over medium heat. Add the curry paste and 2 tablespoons of the coconut milk. Sauté until the oil starts to separate from the curry paste. Add the sweet potatoes, carrots, and onion and to combine. Add the rest of the coconut milk, water, fish sauce, tamarind, and Sucanat. Cook until the potatoes are almost soft (about 15 min.), then add the pepper. Cook until soft. Adjust seasoning to taste.

Note: You can find tamarind juice, fish sauce, and curry paste at an Asian market or the Asian section of the supermarket. They keep forever and are relatively inexpensive. Feel free to experiment with different vegetables - eggplant is also good in this.

Vegetable Minestrone
By: Robert O. and Shelley Redford Young from *The pH Miracle*

Serves 4

1 small cabbage

1 red bell pepper

1 onion

2 carrots

2 celery stalks

2 zucchini

1 yellow summer squash

Flax seed oil, to taste

Bragg Liquid Aminos, to taste

Cayenne pepper, to taste

Cut vegetables as preferred. Cover carrots and celery with water or vegetable broth in soup pot. Cook gently until they just begin to "give" then add remaining vegetables. Do not overcook. Serve hot with flax seed oil, Bragg Liquid Aminos, and cayenne pepper to taste.

SALADS/DRESSING

Spinach Salad I

By: Robert O. and Shelley Redford Young from *The pH Miracle*

I have included the dressing mentioned in this recipe on page 100.

Serves 2-3

1 head spinach

½ cup cauliflower, cut in small pieces

2 stalks celery, chopped

6 radishes, chopped

In a large bowl, combine ingredients and toss well. Top with Essential Dressing (see page 224 of the author's book).

Spinach Salad II

By: Robert O. and Shelley Redford Young from *The pH Miracle*

I have included the dressing mentioned in this recipe on page 100.

Serves 2-3

1 head spinach
½ cup cauliflower, cut in small pieces
2 stalks celery, chopped
6 radishes, chopped
2 shallots, chopped (or 1 small red onion)
½ cup chopped basil
2 red peppers, chopped
4 tablespoons pine nuts

In a large bowl, combine all ingredients and toss well. Top with Essential Dressing (see page 224 of the author's book).

Essential Dressing
By: Robert O. and Shelley Redford Young from *The pH Miracle*

Serves 4-6

1 cup preferred oil (Udo's, Essential Balance, olive, flax seed, or grape seed)
¼ cup Bragg Liquid Aminos or 1 teaspoon Real Salt (adjust to taste)
Juice of 1 fresh lemon
½-1 teaspoon of any seasoning you prefer, such as Italian, Mexican (Spice Hunter), pesto, garlic powder, onion powder, parsley, basil, or oregano

Combine all ingredients in a food processor and mix well or simply place in a salad dressing jar and shake to mix well. Chill and serve.

Tiffany's Ranch Dressing

By Tiffany Perez from *At Tiffany's Table Eat Your Way to Health*

½ cup mayonnaise

½ cup plain yogurt

3 teaspoons raw, apple cider vinegar

3 teaspoons minced onion

1 clove garlic

1 teaspoon fresh oregano, minced

2 teaspoons dried dill

Raw milk, (enough to reach desired thickness)

Sea salt and pepper to taste

Blend all ingredients really well. Best if refrigerated over night.

Strawberry Salad with Orange

By Melissa Chappell from *Faves*

Here is what the originator has to say about it: "One of my very first speaking engagements was for a mama's conference. The committee asked me to present on how to get your kids to eat healthier. I was so excited to be asked to speak, but was a little nervous about creating recipes that would fly with kids. I really, really wanted to send these moms home with something that would be appealing and truly work. This is one of the salads I came up with because kids LOVE strawberries. It also might surprise you how many children will eat greens if they're covered in something really delicious. The presentation ended up being a hit and the women were thrilled to have some healthy and good tasting recipes. Try it on your babies!" She is right my children love this salad.

Serves 4

Salad:

1 head romaine lettuce

1 orange

1 pint strawberries

Dressing:

1 cup frozen strawberries (thawed)

1 tablespoon honey to taste

A splash of balsamic vinegar(optional)

Cut romaine into strips and arrange on 4 plates. Peel, section, and cut oranges into bite size pieces. Slice strawberries. Arrange fruit on top of romaine. Blend all dressing ingredients in a blender. If necessary, add a small amount of water to make blender run smoothly. Pour equal amounts over each salad. You may also toss the salad ingredients and dressing in a bowl to coat and then serve this way. (I like it when all the lettuce in a salad is coated with dressing.)

SIDES

Carrots and Parsnips

By Lauren Hoover-West from recipe book *NO WHEAT, NO DAIRY, NO PROBLEM!* https://nowheatnodairynoproblem.com/cookbook-orders/

Here's what the originator had to say about it: "This is a match made in Heaven, and really good restaurants! As children we all heard, eat your carrots and vegetables...they are good for you! Well, they are good for us, high in antioxidants, and they are delicious when they are not overcooked to mush and seasoned well. Give these a try, and you'll change your mind, and your kids, about vegetables!"

Yields: varies, 1 carrot and 1 parsnip per person
organic carrots
organic parsnips
extra virgin olive oil or grapeseed oil
kosher or sea salt
Pepper grinder
ground cumin in shaker bottle with a shaker top, optional flat leaf parsley, finely chopped, optional

Preheat oven to 400°, if you are really hurried 450° will speed up the cooking. Scrub carrots and parsnips with vegetable wash and rinse well. Leave the peel on the carrots since that is where the most vitamins and minerals are found. Peel the parsnips because the peel can be bitter. Cut off ops and discard. Using a sharp knife and cutting board, cut carrots and parsnips into ½ inch slices, diagonally. Place on a metal baking pan or glass baking dish, but metal will brown better. Drizzle just enough extra virgin olive oil or grapeseed oil to lightly coat them-please no puddles of oil. Sprinkle kosher salt or sea salt and grind black pepper. If you are using cumin, shake it over the carrots and parsnips for a light dusting-this is a very strong spice and should be used in moderation. Bake on the second from the top rack of the oven for approximately 10 minutes. Check by inserting a fork into the carrots and parsnips-if they are soft but still a little resistant or crunchy...they are done. Don't wait for them to be completely soft unless you are going to puree them. Sprinkle fresh chopped parsley over the carrots and parsnips just before serving. Parsley is pretty but also very healthy. I purposely did not include amounts in the recipe because I want to teach you to cook things for various portions. Baking is a different story, and exact measurement is crucial!

Casserole de Cauliflower

By: Robert O. and Shelley Redford Young from *The pH Miracle*

Here is what the originator has to say about it: "Takes 20 minutes to prepare. This dish is a lot like couscous in texture and makes a great breakfast, lunch, or dinner side dish."

Serves 4-6

2 teaspoons oil (olive, flax, or Udo's Choice)

2-4 teaspoons cumin

½ teaspoon turmeric

½ yellow or red onion, finely minced

1 cup water

Florets from 1 very large or 2 small cauliflowers

1 red bell pepper, finely chopped

4 tablespoons fresh parsley, minced

½ cup raw pine nuts

7-8 sun-dried tomatoes (Melissa's brand are packed in olive oil)

Bragg Liquid Aminos, to taste

Lemon or lime juice, to taste

2 cloves of garlic, minced

In an electric skillet, warm the oil, cumin, and turmeric.
Keeping the temperature on warm or low, add the onion and allow the flavors to blend for 2-4 minutes, then add the water and warm. In a food processor fitted with an S-blade, process the cauliflower into very small pieces (like couscous). Also process the sun-dried tomatoes into fine small pieces.
Add the cauliflower to the skillet and gradually warm, adding the parsley, garlic, sun-dried tomatoes, and pine nuts. Season with Bragg Aminos and lemon or lime juice to taste. Enjoy!

Cranberry-Orange Sauce

By: Suzanne Stevens inspired by Rachel Ray

This will change your mind about cranberry sauce as it did mine.

Ingredients:

Zest and juice of 1 orange

1/2 cup raw honey or desired sweetener

Pinch salt

1 12 ounce bag fresh cranberries, rinsed

Directions:

1. In a medium saucepan, combine 1/2 cup water, orange zest, orange juice, honey and salt over medium-high heat, stirring until the sugar dissolves, 2 to 3 minutes.

2. Stir in the cranberries and bring to a boil.

3. Reduce the heat and simmer until the cranberries burst and the sauce has thickened slightly, about 7 minutes.

Let the sauce cool to room temperature before serving.

Leprechaun Surprise Dip

By: Robert O. and Shelley Redford Young from *The pH Miracle*

Serves 6-8

2 cups spinach, very finely chopped

2 cups parsley, very finely chopped

1 cup green onions, very finely chopped

½ cup Mock May (see page 294 of the author's book)

Mix well. Serve with fresh vegetables.

Refried Beans

By: Robert O. and Shelley Redford Young from *The pH Miracle*

Serves 6 (YIELD: 3 CUPS)

3 cups cooked pinto beans
½ cup onion, chopped
1 teaspoon minced garlic
Garlic powder, to taste
Cayenne pepper, to taste
Black pepper, to taste
Real Salt, to taste

Steam fry onions and garlic. Puree pinto beans in food processor or blender. Pour pureed beans into the skillet. Stir beans constantly on low to medium heat until thickened; season while cooking. Serve hot with vegetables.

Smoky Tomato Salsa
By Melissa Chappell from *Faves*

We made this so often I had the recipe memorized and whipped it up whenever surprised guests would arrive.

Here is what the originator has to say about it: "This recipe doesn't need much of an introduction other than to say if you've never had tomato salsa with crushed or toasted cumin seeds in it, you are missing out. The presence of that one ingredient alone gives this salsa a sultry smokiness that won't be lost on anyone who eats it.

makes about 2 cups

3 tomatoes diced
2 green onions thinly sliced
1-2 cloves garlic, minced
1 large handful of cilantro
1 large handful of parsley
1 teaspoon cumin seeds
1 teaspoon salt
1 tablespoon lime juice

Cayenne or crushed red pepper to taste (start with an $\frac{1}{8}$ teaspoon And increase until the salsa reaches the level of heat you like) Smash the cumin seeds with mortar and pestle or chop into small bits with a knife right before adding to bring out the smoky flavor. You may also toast them in a dry pan until browned. Combine all ingredients in a bowl and stir well to integrate the seasonings and get the juices of the tomato flowing. Adjust for seasonings (after this salsa sits for a while the flavors mellow and it may need more salt) and eat.

Savory Green Beans with Tamari

By: Robyn Openshaw & Desiree Ward from *Healthy Holiday Favorites*

This a quite a lovely twist steamed or boiled green beans. I love the garlic flavor. Often I steam green beans and sauté with garlic then salt to taste. You can substitute "Coconut Aminos" from Coconut Secret for the Tamari if desired. It does not change the flavor.

Here is what the originator has to say about it: "Simple and full of flavor, tamari works like a natural probiotic and it is gluten free."

Serves 4-5

2-3 cloves garlic
1 teaspoon extra virgin olive oil
3 cups green beans
¼ cup chopped raw almonds
2 teaspoons tamari

Wash the green beans and trim off the ends. In a large stock pot, bring 2 ½ quarts of water to a rolling boil and generously salt the water. Add the green beans to the boiling water and cook for 3-5 minutes. Drain the water off and rinse the green beans under cold water. In a large frying pan, heat the olive oil over medium heat, then add the garlic and almonds and sauté until golden brown, 3-5 min. Add the green beans and the tamari to the garlic mixture. Cook for about 3-5 min. More until the beans are heated through but slightly crisp. Salt and pepper green beans to taste.

Thai Nut Sauce
By Melissa Chappell from *Faves*

Melissa has a couple of sauces I enjoy from this recipe book. I use this sauce for spring rolls or stir fry. You can substitute "Coconut Aminos" from Coconut Secret for the Tamari if desired. It does not change the flavor.

Here is what the originator has to say about it: "I'm sure hundreds of these cookbooks will sell for this recipe alone. I first introduced this to my private clients and then later added it to a small "lunchbox" line as a dip for veggie spring rolls. The stores got so many requests for the sauce to be sold separately, that now we sell it in the bottles. It really is good as a sauce on everything or as a dip for anything. As one client put it, "You could dip napkins in this sauce and they would taste good!" although I recommend sticking with food."

Makes about 2 cups (see picture on page 76 of the author's book)

1 cup almonds
½ cup olive oil
½ cup tamari sauce
½ cup agave
4 cloves garlic

Blend almonds in a food processor or high-speed blender (a blender will make the sauce smoother) until very fine and flour-like. Add the rest of the ingredients and blend until smooth. Serve this with Spring Rolls, over noodles or rice or as a dip for veggies, steamed or fresh.

Veggie Crunch Stix and Crackers
By: Robert O. and Shelley Redford Young from *The pH Miracle*

Here is what the originator has to say about it: "These colorful snacks are a great way to wean children and adults from yeast breads. They are a wonderful grab-snack and also complement and give crunch to a vegan-based meal such as soup and salad. They work up very fast and travel well. I use the small cookie cutters and make little dinosaurs, airplanes, and heart crackers. Also, you can season them any way you want by adding a couple of teaspoons of your favorite spice."

Serves 8-10

2 cups flour (all-purpose, millet, whole wheat--I use half and half all-purpose and whole wheat)
½-1 teaspoon salt
1 ½ teaspoons baking powder
3 heaping tablespoons soft tofu (Nori brand is good)
2 tablespoons olive oil
1-2 teaspoons Seasonings of your choice (optional)
⅓-¾ cup cold water or fresh vegetable juice, or mix

In a food processor, pulse the flour, the salt, and baking powder to combine. Add the tofu and olive oil and pulse until the mixture resembles coarse meal. With the machine running, gradually add between ½ and ¾ cup ice water or fresh veggie juice until the dough comes together in a soft ball (approximately 1 minute)

Turn the dough out onto a lightly floured surface. Form the dough into a smooth rectangle, about 4 by 6 inches, then roll out the dough into an 8-by-10-inch sheet, ¼ inch thick. With a sharp knife cut the dough lengthwise into ¼-inch-wide strips.

Using your hands, gently roll each strip into 16-inch-long sticks. For a twisted version, grab each end of the dough strip with your fingers and carefully stretch and twist the strip in opposite directions. For crackers use cookie cutters (children love these!) and arrange on baking sheet. Arrange the sticks on two baking sheets, side by side but not touching, and press ends into the baking sheet to keep the sticks straight while they cook. If desired, brush each stick lightly with olive oil and sprinkle with salt or seasonings of your choice. Bae at 350° until firm and cooked through, 14-18 minutes.

Transfer the sticks or crackers to a wire rack to cool. Store in an airtight container at room temperature or two to three days.
Variations:
Beet Stix: 2 tablespoons beet juice, from 1 small beet. Combine with ½ cup cold water.
Popeye Stix: ½ cup parsley or spinach juice. Combine with ¼ cup cold water
Bugs Bunny Stix: ¼ cup carrot juice, from about 3 carrots. Combine with ¼ cup cold water.
Tomato Stix: ¼ cup fresh tomato juice, with 1-2 tablespoons sun-dried tomato pesto. Combine with ⅓ cup cold water.
Spicing Variations:
Curry/Turmeric Stix: 1 teaspoon curry powder, with ½ teaspoon ground turmeric.
Cumin Stix: 2 teaspoons Ground cumin.
Garlic Stix: 2 teaspoons Garlic Herb Bread Seasoning (Spice Hunter)
Mexi Stix: 2 teaspoons Mexican Seasoning (Spice Hunter).
Experiment!

NOTES

As of November 2018 the following web pages and its content are listed below. Corresponding with the section in this book. To learn more read from these below and search other sites not listed.

Step Two: Know ingredients:

How to Read Labeling:
Miriam Levin, "How to Read Food Labels and Avoid Toxic Ingredients", April 12, 2017, Organic Lifestyle Magazine
https://www.organiclifestylemagazine.com/how-to-read-food-labels-and-avoid-toxic-ingredients

Oils:
Dr. Mark Hyman, "Why Oil is Bad for You", DrHyman.com
https://drhyman.com/blog/2016/01/29/why-oil-is-bad-for-you/

Robin Konie, "The ugly truth about vegetable oils (and why they should be avoided), Thank Your Body
https://www.thankyourbody.com/vegetable-oils/

"Good Fats VS. Bad Fats: Dr. Hy,aman's Healthy Cheat Sheet", The Chalkboard
http://thechalkboardmag.com/dr-hyman-good-fat-bad-fat

Dr. Chris Kresser, "The Truth About Fat with Chris Kresser", Paleohacks
https://blog.paleohacks.com/the-truth-about-fat-with-chris-kresser/

Hidden sugars:
University of California San Francisco, sugarscience the unsweetened truth, "Hidden in Plain Sight"
http://sugarscience.ucsf.edu/hidden-in-plain-sight/#.W1zPjdhKgQ8

Annette McDermott, Certified in Food, Nutrition and Health, "Other Names for Sugar on Food Labels", LoveToKnow
https://diet.lovetoknow.com/wiki/
Other_Names_for_Sugar_on_Food_Labels

Catherine Saxelby, "48 shades of hidden sugars!", July 6, 2016, Foodwatch
https://foodwatch.com.au/blog/carbs-sugars-and-fibres/item/48-shades-of-hidden-sugars.html

Sugar replacements:
Dr. Josh Axe, "5 Best Sugar Substitutes", November 21, 2015, Dr. Axe,
https://draxe.com/sugar-substitutes/

Lauren Hoover-West, "Coconut Palm Sugar-Low Glycemic Index sugar alternative!", August, 21, No Wheat, No Dairy, No Problem!
https://nowheatnodairynoproblem.com/2009/08/21/coconut-palm-sugar-low-glycemic-index-sugar-alternative/

Agave:
Referencing Agave as unhealthy:

PubMed, "Effect of moderate intake of sweeteners on metabolic health in the rat.", December 7, 2009, Figlewicz DP, Ioannou G, Bennett Jay J, Kittleson S, Savard C, Roth CL,
https://www.ncbi.nlm.nih.gov/pubmed/19815021

PubMed, "Total antioxidant content of alternative to refined sugar.", January 2009, Phillips KM, Carlsen NH, Blomhoff R,
https://www.ncbi.nlm.nih.gov/pubmed/19103324

PubMed, "Saponions of Agave: Chemistry and bioactivity." October 2016, Sidana J, Singh B, Sharma OP,
https://www.ncbi.nlm.nih.gov/pubmed/27374482

The OZ Blog, "Agave: Why WE Were Wrong", Mehmet Pz, MD, http://blog.doctoroz.com/dr-oz-blog/agave-why-we-were-wrong Merola Take Control of Your. Health, "Shocking! The "Tequila" Sweetner Agave Is Far Worse Than High Fructose Corn Syrup", March 30, 2000, Dr. Joseph Mercola
 https://articles.mercola.com/sites/articles/archive/2010/03/30/ beware-of-the-agave-nectar-health-food.aspx#_edn1

Huffington Post"Debunking The Blue Agave Myth, Agave nectar syrup is a triumph of marketing over science.", April 17, 2010, Dr. Johnny Bowden, Contributor
https://www.huffpost.com/entry/debunking-the-blue-agave_b_450144

Referencing Agave as healthy:
http://wholesomesweet.com/faqs/agave-fact-vs-fiction/

Oils replacements:
Rachael Link, MS, RD, "11 Best Healthy Fats for Your Body", July 25, 2018, Dr. Axe
https://draxe.com/healthy-fats/

"Good Fats VS. Bad Fats: Dr. Hy,aman's Healthy Cheat Sheet", The Chalkboard
http://thechalkboardmag.com/dr-hyman-good-fat-bad-fat

Michael Ravensthorpe, "What are the healthiest cooking oils?", May 31, 2015, Natural News
https://www.naturalnews.com/ 049901_cooking_oils_coconut_oil_olive.html

Preservatives:
James Colquhoun, "22 Additives And Preservatives To Avoid", November 1, 2016, Food Matters
https://www.foodmatters.com/article/22-additives-and-preservatives-to-avoid

Step Four: Salt
Dr. Brownstein, "Salt, Your Way to Health", Dr. Brownstein's Holistic Medicine
https://www.drbrownstein.com/salt-your-way-to-health-p/salt.htm

Dr. Brownstein, "Lower Your Salt Intake? Fugetaboutit!", August 15, 2014, Dr. Brownstein's Holistic Medicine
https://www.drbrownstein.com/lower-your-salt-intake-fugetaboutit/

Dr. Brownstein, "Why Salt is GOOD For You and 5 Healthy Ways To Use It", March 24, 2014, Dr. Brownstein's Holistic Medicine
https://www.drbrownstein.com/why-salt-is-good-for-you-5-healthy-ways-to-use-it-2/

Step Eight: Water
Dr. F. Batmanghelidj, The Water Cure
http://www.watercure.com/

Institute of Medicine of the National Academies, The National Academies Press and the Transportation Research Board, Free PDF version
https://www.nap.edu/catalog/10925/dietary-reference-intakes-for-water-potassium-sodium-chloride-and-sulfate

Step Nine: Meats
Kristen Michaelis, "Healthy Meats:What to Buy", Food Renegade
https://www.foodrenegade.com/healthy-meats-what-to-buy/

Anthony Gustin, "Source Matters: A Guide to Buying Healthy Meats", Dr. Anthony Gustin
http://www.dranthonygustin.com/guide-healthy-meats/Recipes:

Sandra Ramcher, "Healing Foods Cooking for Celiacs, Colitis, Crohn's and IBS"
 https://healingfoodscookbook.com/healing-foods/

Robyn Openshaw & Desiree Ward , "Healthy Holiday Favorites"
https://shop.greensmoothiegirl.com/products/healthy-holiday-favorites

By: Robyn Openshaw , "The Green Smoothies Diet"
https://shop.greensmoothiegirl.com/products/green-smoothies-diet

Tiffany Perez, "At Tiffany's Table Eat Your Way to Health"
https://www.amazon.com/Tiffanys-Table-Eat-Your-Health/dp/156684701X?
keywords=at+tiffany%27s+table+book&qid=1540606646&sr=8-3&ref=sr_1_3

http://store.alpineclinic.net/product/at-tiffany-s-table/

Melissa Chappell, "Faves"
https://freshmelissa.com/shop/faves-cookbook/

Robert O. and Shelley Redford Young , "The pH Miracle"
For information on Dr. Robert O Young: www.drrobertyoung.com
Books: www.phoreveryoung.com
Dr. Young pH Miracle Retreats: www.phmiracleretreat.com

Cover Photo:
Max Pixel, https://www.maxpixel.net/Fruit-Delicious-Strawberries-Berries-Food-Eat-3431122

LEARN NUTRITION - BECOME A HEALTH COACH

This book was inspired by my experience at the Institute for Integrative Nutrition® (IIN), where I received my training in holistic wellness and health coaching.

IIN offers a truly comprehensive Health Coach Training Program that invites students to deeply explore the things that are most nourishing to them. From the physical aspects of nutrition and eating wholesome foods that work best for each individual person, to the concept of Primary Food – the idea that everything in life, including our spirituality, career, relationships, and fitness contributes to our inner and outer health – IIN helped me reach optimal health and balance. This inner journey unleashed the passion that compels me to share what I've learned and inspire others.

Beyond personal health, IIN offers training in health coaching, as well as business and marketing. Students who choose to pursue this field professionally complete the program equipped with the communication skills and branding knowledge they need to create a fulfilling career encouraging and supporting others in reaching their own health goals.

From renowned wellness experts as Visiting Teachers to the convenience of their online learning platform, this school has changed my life, and I believe it will do the same for you. I invite you to learn more about the Institute for Integrative Nutrition and explore how the Health Coach Training Program can help you transform your life. Feel free to contact me to hear more about my personal experience at www.SuzyCooking.com/integrative-nutrition, or call (844) 315-8546 to learn more.

ABOUT THE AUTHOR

In high school, Suzanne Stevens' career of choice was to be a mother, though wanting to go to college and get an education before getting married and starting her family. She attended Ricks College (now Brigham Young University - Idaho) and received her degree in Information Management because of her love in computers, a perfect match for her husband, Robert, who is a Computer Scientist/Entrepreneur. He has been a wonderful provider during their twenty-nine years of marriage.

As a stay-at-home mother of seven, she took her family through a transition to better health while trying to heal her acid reflux. Since her transformation, she enjoys nutrition and helping others do the same.

She never considered going back to school until one day she received an impression to get a nutrition degree. After research, she decided to attend the Institute for Integrative Nutrition® (IIN). She chose this school because it was in line with what she was learning, practicing, and because some of the visiting teachers were doctors and others she has been learning from on her own.

Suzanne enjoys reading to her children, cooking, crocheting, doing crafts, reading a good book, watching movies, being outdoors, and exercising.

www.ingramcontent.com/pod-product-compliance
Lightning Source LLC
Chambersburg PA
CBHW061812250726
48657CB00001B/394